Color Atlas of
CORNEAL DYSTROPHIES
AND DEGENERATIONS

Color Atlas of
CORNEAL DYSTROPHIES AND DEGENERATIONS

Thomas A. Casey
MCh, FRCS, FCOphth
Consultant Ophthalmic Surgeon
Director, Corneo-Plastic Unit and National Eye Bank
Queen Victoria Hospital
East Grinstead
England

Khaled W. Sharif
FRCS, FCOphth
Fellow in Corneal Surgery
Corneo-Plastic Unit and National Eye Bank
Queen Victoria Hospital
East Grinstead
England

Head, Department of Ophthalmology
University of Jordan
Faculty of Medicine
Amman

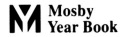
Mosby
Year Book

St. Louis   Baltimore   Boston   Chicago   London   Philadelphia   Sydney   Toronto

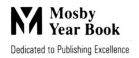

Mosby–Year Book, Inc.
11830 Westline Drive
St. Louis, MO 63146

Copyright © 1991 Wolfe Publishing Ltd.
All rights reserved.
Published in 1991 with rights in the USA, Canada and Puerto Rico by
Mosby–Year Book, Inc.

ISBN 0–8151–1445–1

English edition first published by Wolfe Publishing Ltd.
2–16 Torrington Place, London WC1E 7LT, UK.

Library of Congress Cataloging-in-Publication Data has been applied for.

Contents

Acknowledgements

We are very grateful to Mrs Susan Forbes for her great help in typing
the manuscript before presentation to the publishers. Those colleagues
who referred their patients to us must be remembered, but our
special thanks go to the patients themselves for providing
the real material for this Atlas.

Preface

Corneal dystrophies and degenerations present a bewildering range of features, as many ophthalmologists-in-training soon discover in their search for the right diagnostic labels; such confusion is indeed familiar to more established ophthalmologists, whose patients are apt to ask taxing questions about the natural history and course of the disease, and the prognosis after grafting. It is true that detailed descriptions are readily available in textbooks, but they are often hard to relate to the accompanying pictures, which are usually in black and white, few in number, and all too often bear little relationship to the cases we actually see in the clinic.

Consequently, in this Atlas, we provide in large format a series of high-quality colour photographs and paintings that display the specific features of most of the dystrophies and degenerations that may be encountered. We do not intend our book to be used in isolation, but hope that it will prove useful in conjunction with the comprehensive (albeit sparsely illustrated) textbooks on corneal disease that are already available.

Nearly all the cases that we have presented were patients examined and followed up in our corneal and external eye diseases clinics; this has allowed us to provide photographic evidence of the early signs and the progression of the various dystrophies, and to examine the families of our patients, enabling us to demonstrate any hereditary patterns, together with the variations in their clinical presentation.

We hope that this Atlas will resolve some of the diagnostic difficulties, and that it will take its place as a welcome source of reference.

TA Casey
KW Sharif

Dedication

This book is dedicated to our families.

1 Anterior corneal dystrophies

Hereditary epithelial dystrophy (Meesmann's)

Meesmann's dystrophy is a rare, bilateral, and symmetrical disorder of the corneal epithelium, with an autosomal dominant pattern of inheritance. First described by Pomeijer in 1935, the condition was more comprehensively documented by Meesmann and Wilke three years later. It may present in the first year of life as epithelial microcysts that are only visible by slit-lamp magnification. Patients remain asymptomatic until early adult life or middle age, when the cysts begin to rupture, causing recurrent corneal erosions that clinically produce intermittent attacks of pain and photophobia. In most cases, there is no impairment of visual acuity and the affected patients are only periodically symptomatic. However, recurrent episodes of corneal erosions may lead to the development of subepithelial scarring and irregular astigmatism.

Slit-lamp examination is essential in making the diagnosis. Multiple, fine, round cysts are detectable in the epithelium. They are most prominent in the interpalpebral zone, although they can eventually involve the whole corneal surface as their number and density increase throughout life. On retroillumination, these lesions take on the appearance of fine vesicles that are regular in size and shape. Coalescence of the cysts may form refractile clusters or lines. In advanced cases, serpiginous grey lines and small amorphous subepithelial opacities may be seen in addition to the characteristic microcysts.

In hereditary epithelial dystrophy, light microscopy demonstrates a diffusely disorganised epithelial layer of variable thickness, with cytoplasmic vacuolation. Small, round, debris-filled intraepithelial cysts, ranging from 10–100 µm, are found throughout the epithelial layers, most prominently in the anterior third. Electron microscopy reveals a material described as 'peculiar substance' within the epithelial cells, most characteristically in the basal layers. The dystrophy appears to be a primary result of the accumulation of this material within the cells, with secondary changes in the form of increased cell turnover, thickened basement membrane, and cell degeneration.

Treatment is seldom required, as visual loss is extremely rare. Lamellar or penetrating keratoplasty may be indicated in a few selected cases with advanced subepithelial scarring.

1 Meesmann's dystrophy in a 25-year-old asymptomatic patient. On retroillumination, the microcysts appear as multiple, fine, clear intra-epithelial vesicles. On direct focal illumination, they appear as discrete, grey dots. Note the typical distribution of these vesicles, being more concentrated at the central interpalpebral cornea.

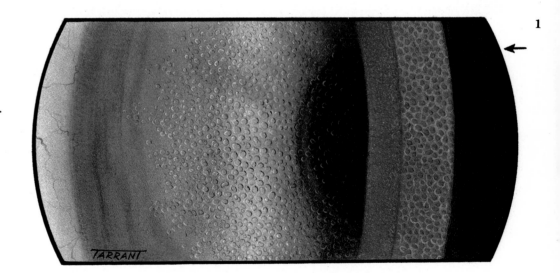

1

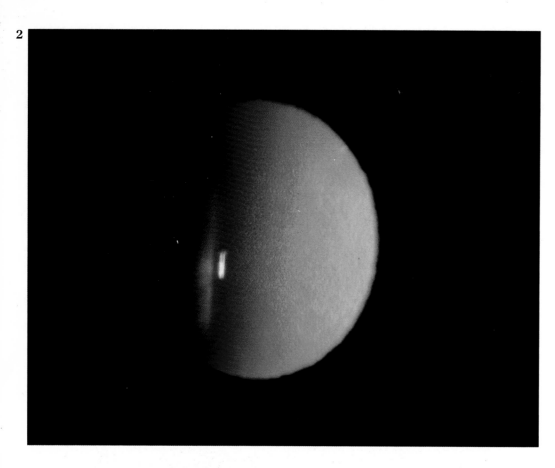

2 Retroillumination following pupillary dilatation can be very useful in demonstrating the extent and the distribution of the epithelial microcysts. In this patient, there was peripheral, as well as central, corneal involvement. The patient's father and sister had similar corneal epithelial changes, confirming the autosomal dominant inheritance pattern of the dystrophy. All the affected members of the family had normal visual acuity and were only intermittently symptomatic.

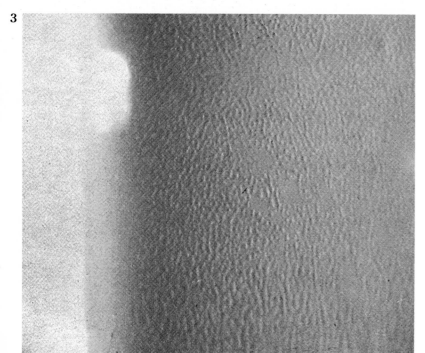

3 High-magnification slit-lamp photograph of the fellow eye of the patient in **2**. There is a similar pattern, with diffuse distribution of the fine vesicles. Note that these vesicles are of uniform size and shape, and that the intervening cornea is clear. These microcysts differ from those seen in Cogan's dystrophy, in that they are not white, are more vesicular, more uniform in size and shape, and more diffusely distributed.

Epithelial basement membrane dystrophy (Cogan's)

Epithelial basement membrane dystrophy (also called map–dot–fingerprint dystrophy) is the most common anterior corneal dystrophy. It was first described by Cogan in 1964, but no recognised hereditary pattern has yet been identified. The pattern of familial occurrence originally suggested an autosomal dominant inheritance. However, several recent studies have identified the map–dot–fingerprint abnormalities in a large percentage of the asymptomatic general population.

The pathogenesis of this dystrophy is related to the primary synthesis of an abnormal epithelial basement membrane with intraepithelial extensions. These extensions block the normal maturation and desquamation of the underlying epithelial cells, with subsequent degeneration of the cells, and focal collections of cellular debris.

On slit-lamp examination, there may be dots, maps, fingerprint opacities, or a combination of these patterns. The most frequently encountered and probably the earliest change in epithelial basement membrane dystrophy is the map-like pattern. The 'maps', which are highlighted by retroillumination, are circumscribed areas with a ground-glass appearance at the centre, and sharply demarcated margins. The 'dots' are fine, grey-white opacities which may be round, oblong, or comma-shaped. The 'fingerprint' lines are the least frequently encountered of the characteristic changes, and are best seen by retroillumination. In addition to the typical triad of map, dot, and fingerprint patterns, there may be other configurations, such as 'blebs' or 'nets'. However, neither blebs nor nets alone disrupt the corneal surface.

Most affected individuals remain asymptomatic throughout life, but some patients may present with symptoms of recurrent corneal erosions, typically when they reach their thirties. These episodes usually occur spontaneously or may be precipitated by minor trauma. The development of the erosions is attributed to the poor epithelial adhesion to the underlying abnormal basement membrane. Although these erosions diminish in frequency with time, the use of topical 5% sodium chloride drops during the day and a similar hypertonic ointment at night may be required to reduce the epithelial oedema and the recurrence of the erosions.

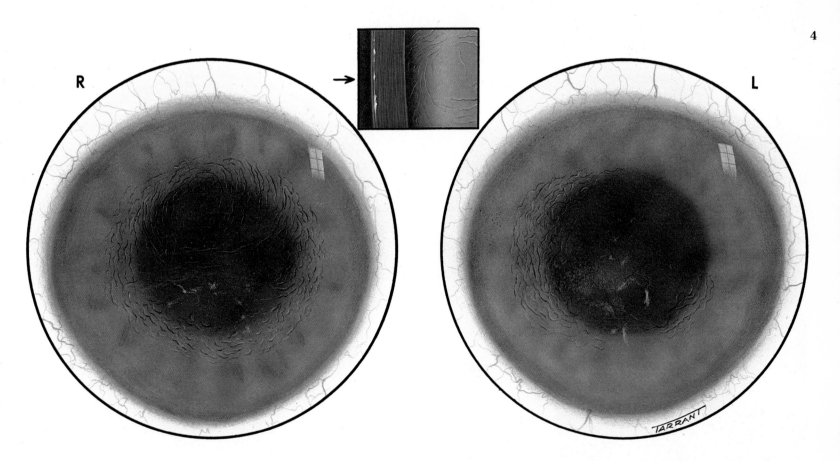

4 Bilateral epithelial basement membrane dystrophy in a 53-year-old woman. Note the 'fingerprint' pattern, together with the grey-white epithelial dots. The left cornea shows associated central subepithelial scarring that has developed secondary to the recurrent episodes of corneal erosions.

5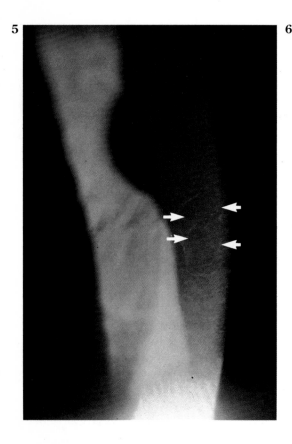

6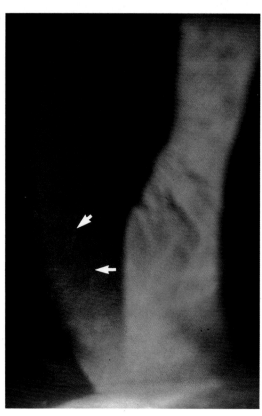

5 & 6 The map-like pattern is clearly evident in both corneas of this patient (arrows). These lesions are best seen by broad oblique illumination, and appear as a superficial, geographic haze interrupted by clear areas, the margins of which are well demarcated. When fluorescein is applied to the corneal surface overlying the 'map', negative staining is detected over the elevated areas. The 'maps' can range in size from several hundred microns to areas covering several square millimetres of corneal surface.

7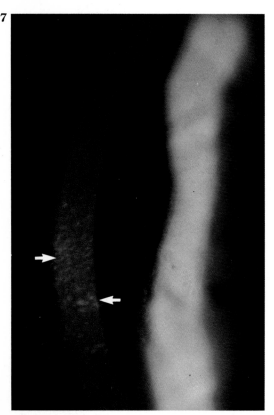

7 The 'dot' pattern of Cogan's dystrophy is also seen in the left eye of the patient in **5 & 6**. Note the fine, grey, dot-like epithelial lesions (arrows), which vary in size and shape. This patient suffered from painful recurrent epithelial erosions that occurred over a period of five years, with spontaneous improvement and no significant effect on visual acuity.

8 Areas of negative staining with fluorescein (arrows) are demonstrated in the same patient as shown in **7**. This finding is related to the irregularity of the pre-corneal tear film overlying the areas affected by the dystrophy.

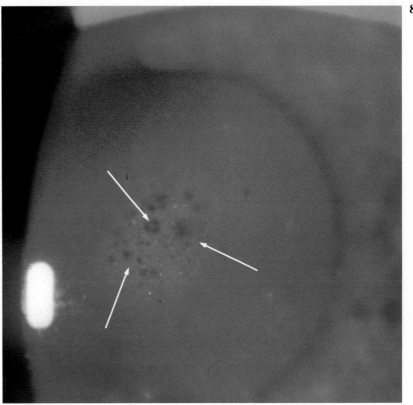

9 'Fingerprint' lines in epithelial basement membrane dystrophy appear as multiple, refractile ridges, best seen by retroillumination. These lines are situated, in most cases, in the central or midperipheral cornea, frequently surrounding the 'maps'. Some may appear as cylindrical processes that may branch, while others have club-shaped terminations. 'Mares' tails' and 'tram lines' are also variants of 'fingerprints', with characteristic aggregate morphologies (Courtesy of British Journal of Ophthalmology).

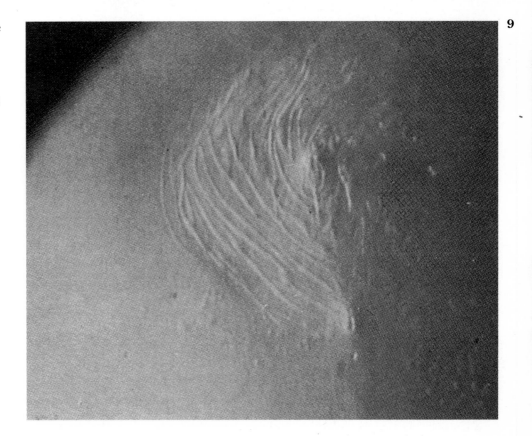

Reis–Bücklers' dystrophy

Reis–Bücklers' dystrophy is a bilateral disorder with symmetrical involvement of the central cornea. It was first clearly described by Reis in 1917, and Bücklers subsequently detailed the clinical picture, documenting the dominant inheritance and strong penetrance.

The disorder presents during early childhood, in the form of fine, reticular opacification at the level of Bowman's layer, which is the earliest slit-lamp finding. The affected child typically complains of recurrent episodes of ocular irritation and photophobia caused by corneal epithelial erosions. Initially, there is only a transient impairment of visual acuity. However, as the dystrophy develops, progressive visual loss occurs due to anterior corneal opacification and irregular astigmatism.

Up to the age of 30 years, Bowman's layer gradually becomes replaced by scar tissue, with a subsequent decrease in the frequency of the acute erosion episodes. The pain experienced during the attacks of erosion becomes greatly diminished, as a direct result of the decrease in corneal sensation. Slit-lamp examination of advanced cases shows marked irregularity of the corneal surface, best seen with a narrow slit-lamp beam. The characteristic discrete, bluish-white, subepithelial opacities, which take a variety of forms, are most dense in the central or midperipheral parts of the cornea, whereas the extreme periphery almost always remains clear. However, on retroillumination, a fine, diffuse haze usually extends to the limbus.

Light microscopy confirms the varying thickness of the epithelial layer which gives it a 'sawtooth' configuration. Many epithelial cells, especially those in the basal layers, demonstrate cytoplasmic vacuolation, mitochondrial swelling, and clumping of nuclear chromatin. Bowman's layer is almost totally replaced by an eosinophilic, PAS-positive material that appears stratified and which may project into the epithelium. Similar material may also be present in the anterior stroma.

Electron microscopy of this subepithelial layer demonstrates closely packed collagen fibrils with a diameter of 300–400 Å and normal periodicity, interspersed with clumps and sheets of short, half-moon-shaped, tubular microfibrils with a diameter of 100 Å. The cause and nature of these characteristic fibrils remain unclear. It is believed that Reis–Bücklers' dystrophy is primarily a Bowman's layer disorder, with resultant secondary basement membrane and epithelial changes. Other theories include primary epithelial, epithelial basement membrane, and neurotrophic causes.

Advanced cases, with marked impairment of vision, have been treated with lamellar or penetrating keratoplasty. However, recurrence of the dystrophy in the grafts is well recognised, and repeat grafting may be indicated in many cases. Excimer laser has also proved to be very effective in treating selected cases with Reis–Bücklers' dystrophy.

10

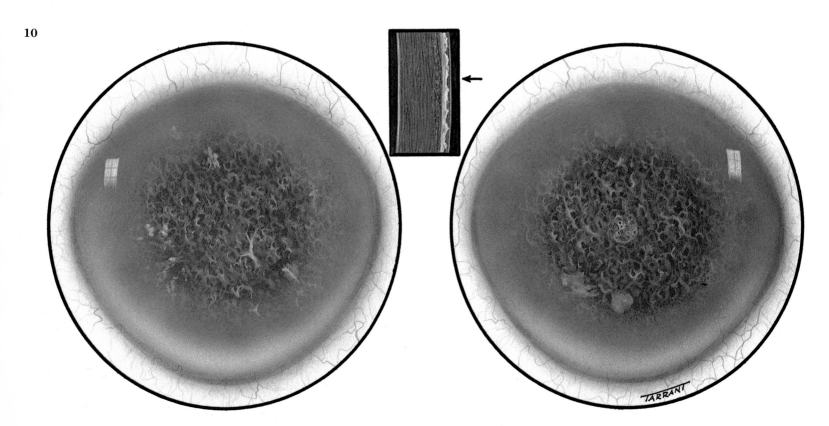

10 Reis–Bücklers' dystrophy in a 25-year-old patient. Note the bilateral and symmetrical corneal lesion at the level of Bowman's layer, with anteriorly projecting ridges into the epithelium. The dystrophy had been documented in four generations of this patient's family.

Progression of Reis–Bücklers' dystrophy

11 The earliest slit-lamp finding in Reis–Bücklers' dystrophy is fine reticular opacification at the level of Bowman's layer, seen here in a 14-year-old boy who presented with a history of recurrent ocular irritation and photophobia. The overall pattern of the lesions is best seen by broad oblique illumination.

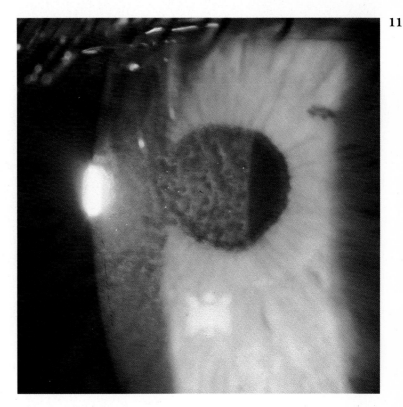

12 A narrow slit-lamp beam demonstrates the anterior location of the opacities, together with the related irregularity of the corneal surface. The acute erosive episodes of this patient diminished in frequency over a period of 10 years. When this photograph was taken, his slit-lamp findings were stable and his corneal sensation had diminished.

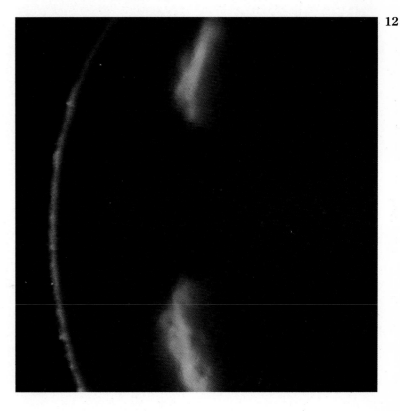

13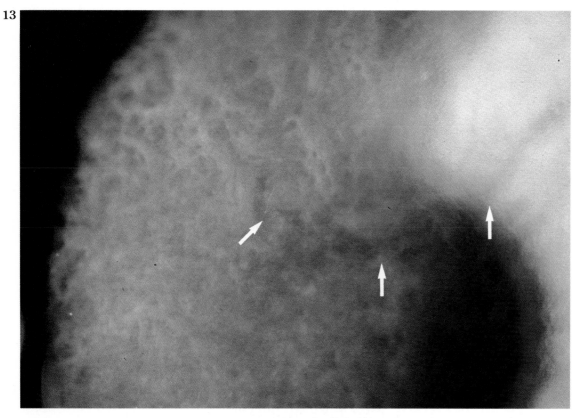

A more advanced case of Reis–Bücklers' dystrophy than that shown on **12**. Note that the greyish white subepithelial opacities have taken a variety of forms. Some are linear, while others have a ring-like, honeycomb, or alveolar pattern. A Hudson–Stähli line (arrows) is commonly seen in advanced cases. The mechanism of formation of this pigment line is related to the associated irregularity of the corneal surface, which subsequently leads to disturbance of the pre-corneal tear film; pooling of the tears at certain areas results, followed by iron deposition in the basal layers of the corneal epithelium.

14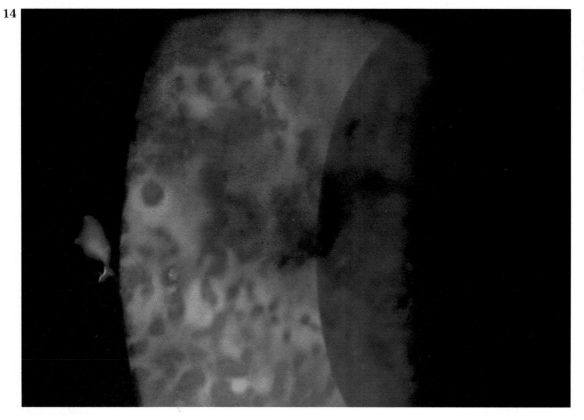

The irregularity of the corneal surface, which is caused by the variable thickness of the epithelial layer, can lead to irregular astigmatism. Negative fluorescein staining is revealed by examination with cobalt-blue light.

15 Light microscopy confirms the varying thickness of the epithelial layer. Bowman's layer, which is fragmented, has been partially replaced by an eosinophilic material that appears stratified and can be seen projecting into the epithelium. Inflammatory changes are absent (Van Gieson's stain × *20*). Loss of hemidesmosomes and disordered basement membrane complexes were demonstrated in this case by electron microscopy. The posterior stroma, Descemet's membrane, and endothelium are normal.

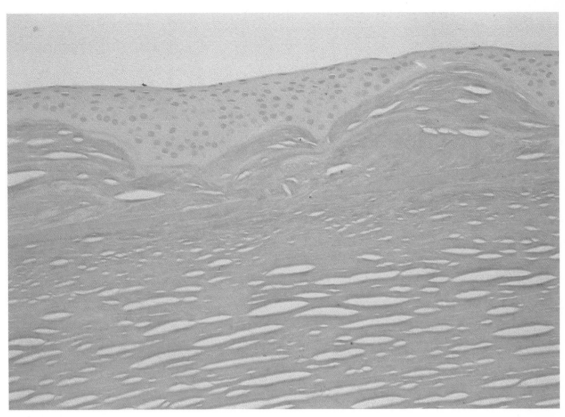

16 Early recurrence of Reis–Bücklers' dystrophy 18 months after penetrating keratoplasty had been performed. Note that the subepithelial recurrence has developed at the periphery of the donor cornea near the graft–host junction, and that it is extending towards the centre. The patient was asymptomatic, and his best corrected visual acuity was 6/6.

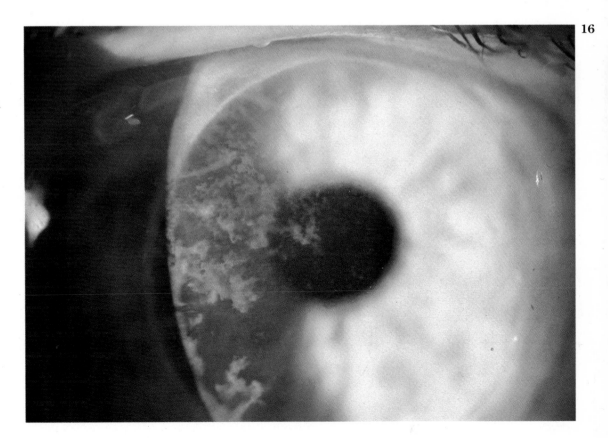

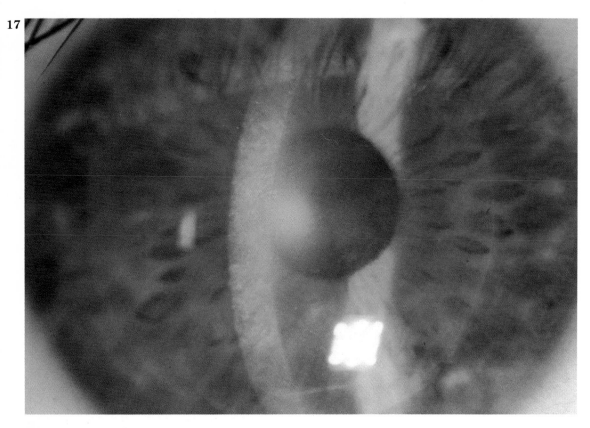

17 A more advanced recurrence of Reis–Bücklers' dystrophy, four years after penetrating keratoplasty. Best corrected visual acuity was 6/18. Note the fine, reticular opacification at the centre of the graft.

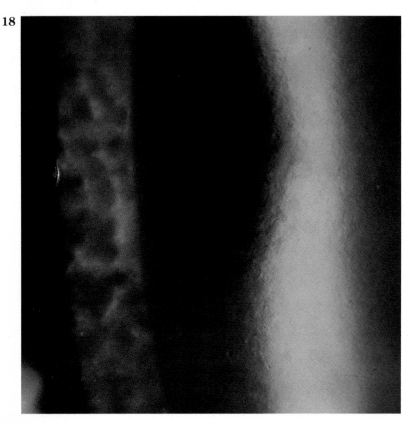

18 High-magnification slit-lamp photograph of the eye shown in **17**. Note that the recurrent lesion has assumed the same honeycomb pattern that was present in the original host cornea preoperatively. Progression of this superficial opacification continued over the following two years, with a further drop in visual acuity to 6/36. Visual rehabilitation was achieved by a repeat penetrating keratoplasty.

Anterior membrane dystrophy (Grayson–Wilbrandt)

An autosomal dominant disorder, first described by Grayson and Wilbrandt in 1966, anterior membrane dystrophy is relatively rare and has a clinical picture similar to that of Reis–Bücklers' dystrophy.

Both dystrophies involve the anterior cornea, and the clinical onset, which occurs during the first ten years of life, takes the form of recurrent corneal erosions. However, anterior membrane dystrophy differs from Reis–Bücklers' dystrophy in the following ways:

- The episodes of recurrent corneal erosion are much less frequent.
- Visual acuity is less severely affected.
- Corneal sensation remains normal.
- Corneal involvement is mainly central, with sparing of the peripheral cornea.
- The anterior cornea intervening between the characteristic lesions remains clear.

Slit-lamp examination reveals characteristic epithelial basement membrane and subepithelial changes, in the form of grey-white, amorphous opacities of varying sizes over the central cornea. These opacities consist of mounds that extend into the epithelium from a thickened Bowman's layer. Light microscopy shows a PAS-positive subepithelial material extending into the basal epithelial layers. Bowman's layer is either absent or replaced by this material. Electron microscopy demonstrates thickening or focal loss of the epithelial basement membrane, and a lack of hemidesmosomes.

19 Anterior membrane dystrophy in a 35-year-old woman. Oblique slit-lamp illumination demonstrates grey-white, amorphous subepithelial opacities of varying size and shape in the central cornea (arrows). Note that the intervening stroma is relatively clear.

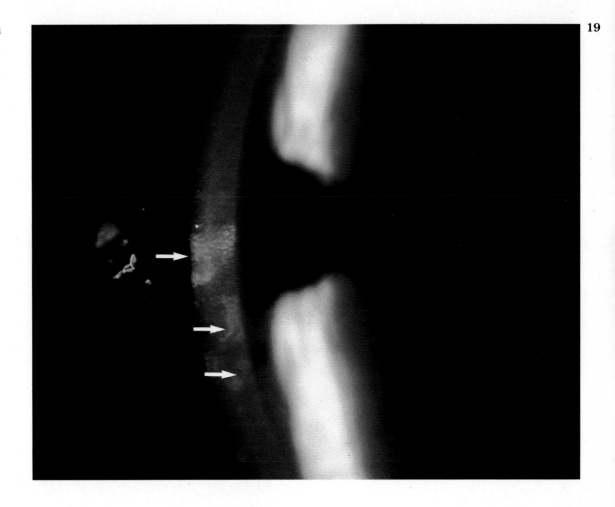

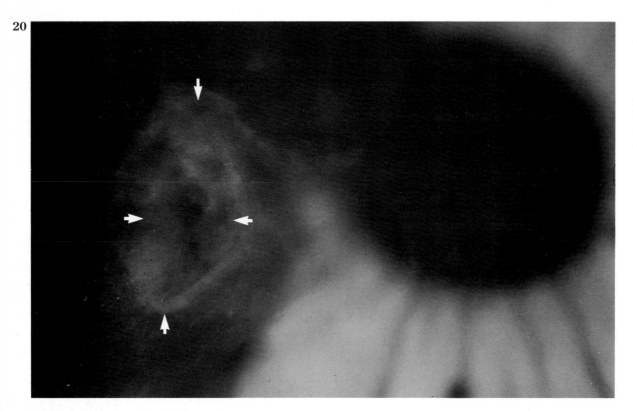

20 High-magnification slit-lamp photograph of one of the sub-epithelial opacities seen in **19** (arrows). The presenting symptoms of this patient were recurrent attacks of ocular irritation and photophobia due to episodes of corneal epithelial erosions.

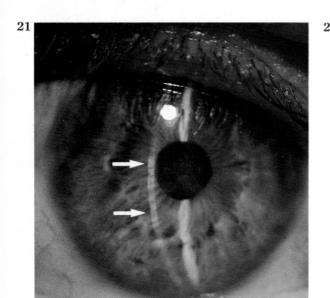

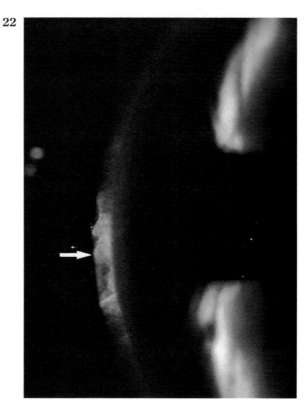

21 & 22 The father of the patient seen in **19 & 20** had similar dystrophic changes, manifested by greyish white subepithelial lesions located in the centre of both corneas (arrows). However, these opacities were less prominent than the lesions found in his daughter, and he was completely asymptomatic.

2 Stromal dystrophies

Lattice dystrophy

Lattice dystrophy is a stromal dystrophy that has an autosomal dominant inheritance pattern. The expression of the gene is often so subtle that the disease can be detected in only a few members of an affected family. The dystrophy, of which there are two types, usually presents in the first decade of life, with symptoms of recurrent erosions or visual disturbance. Less typically, the clinical and symptomatic onset occurs in the fourth decade or later. Lattice dystrophy type I is the classic type with no systemic involvement, while type II is associated with systemic amyloidosis that can involve various organs, as well as the skin of the eyelids and the lacrimal gland.

The characteristic early findings include anterior refractive stromal dots, fine lines, and subepithelial white spots. The translucent lattice lines slowly develop into larger, thicker, more radially oriented lines with a ropy appearance. The stroma intervening between them is clear early in the course of the disease, but becomes progressively more hazy. It is this progressive stromal clouding, together with the scarring caused by recurrent erosions, that eventually leads to a marked reduction in vision. Decreased central corneal sensation occurs by the third decade of life, and the patient may become symptomatically stable.

The deposits in lattice dystrophy are amyloid, demonstrating characteristic staining with Congo red, and manifesting green birefringence when viewed with the polarising microscope. Systemic amyloidosis may be associated with lattice dystrophy type II, which is characterised by fewer lattice lines (than type I) that involve mainly the peripheral cornea, with relative central sparing.

Recurrence of the dystrophy following penetrating keratoplasty occurs more commonly than in other stromal dystrophies, and usually becomes clinically evident after periods ranging from three to 26 years.

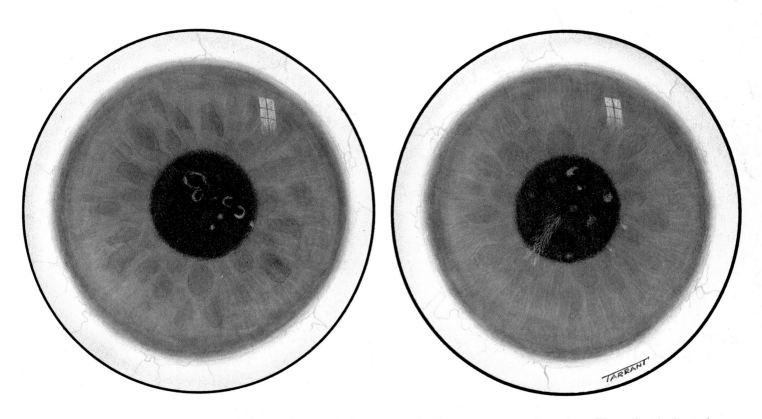

23 Bilateral early lattice dystrophy in an eight-year-old girl who presented with recurrent corneal erosions. The patient had anterior stromal, refractile dots. Her mother had classic lattice dystrophy.

24 High-magnification slit-lamp photograph of the eye shown in **23**. Note the presence of typical anterior stromal, glassy, homogeneous, refractile dots. No lattice lines were detected at this early stage. The presence of stromal dots without accompanying lattice lines in early lattice dystrophy may lead to diagnostic difficulties. However, the clarity of the intervening stroma, and the characteristic glassy appearance of the dots both help to distinguish early lattice dystrophy from other stromal dystrophies.

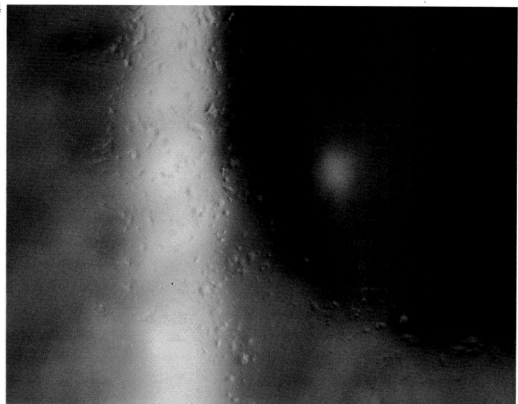

25 The same patient as shown in **23 & 24**, two years later. Note the early appearance of lattice lines (arrows), surrounded by the previously detected refractile dots.

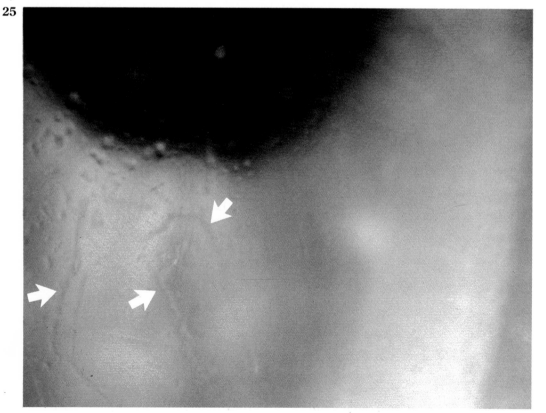

26 & 27 Typical lattice lines are best seen by retroillumination. Note their radial orientation and dichotomous branching. The associated anterior stromal haze (arrow) is also visible. With higher magnification (**27**), the lattice lines appear as double contoured, glassy rods with optically clear cores.

26

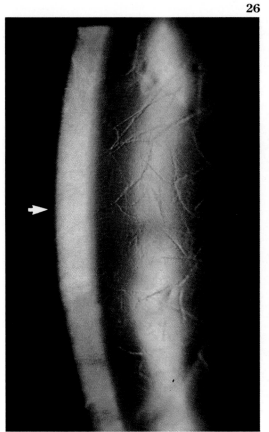

27

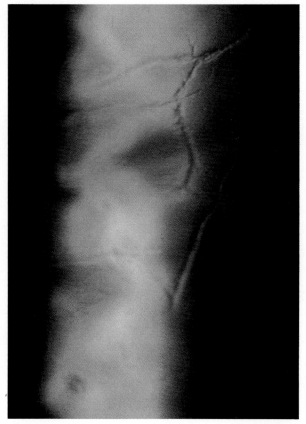

28 Lattice lines fluoresce under cobalt-blue slit-lamp illumination, as seen in this advanced case. This 35-year-old patient had a history of recurrent corneal erosions involving both eyes since he was 10 years old. Both his brother and his sister experienced similar corneal changes.

28

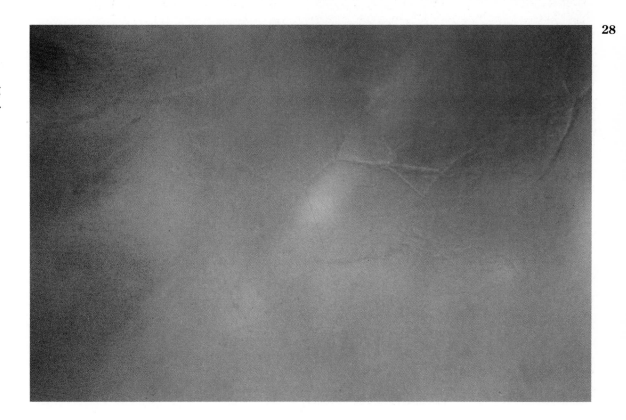

29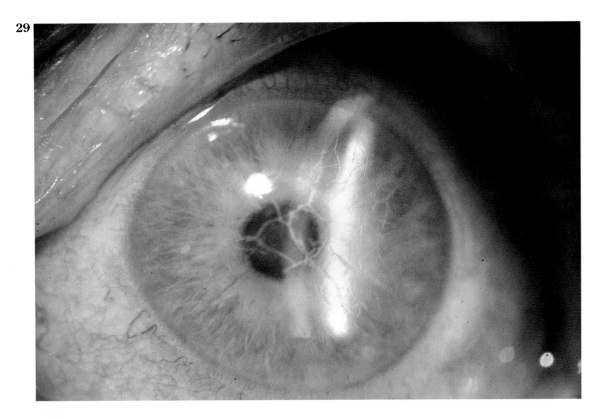

29 As the dystrophy progresses, the lattice lines become thicker and more opaque. With time, the lines become fewer and less distinct, with a ropy appearance.

30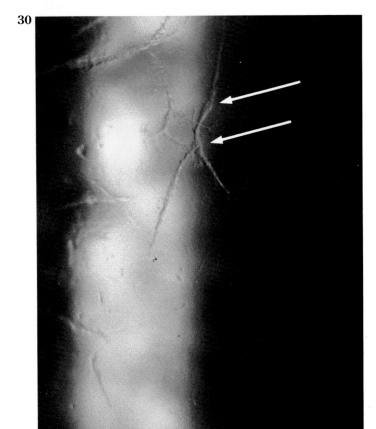

30 Lattice lines in advanced cases can show localised nodular dilatation (arrows), best seen by retroillumination.

31 A more advanced case than that in **30**, showing coarse lattice bands, with nodular dilatation and stromal haze. Best corrected visual acuity was 6/36. These coarse bands constitute a characteristic slit-lamp finding of advanced stages of lattice dystrophy. Following penetrating keratoplasty, visual rehabilitation was achieved in this patient.

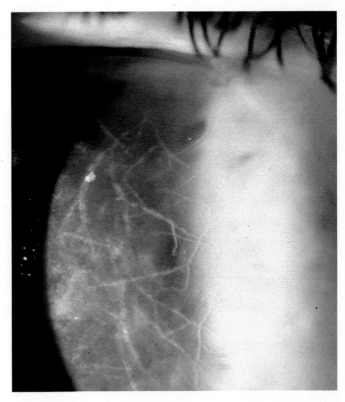

32 Central subepithelial scarring due to recurrent erosions in a 35-year-old woman with lattice dystrophy. These subepithelial opacities may be confused with Reis–Bücklers' dystrophy. However, the presence of the typical branching, refractile lines (arrows) confirms the diagnosis of lattice dystrophy.

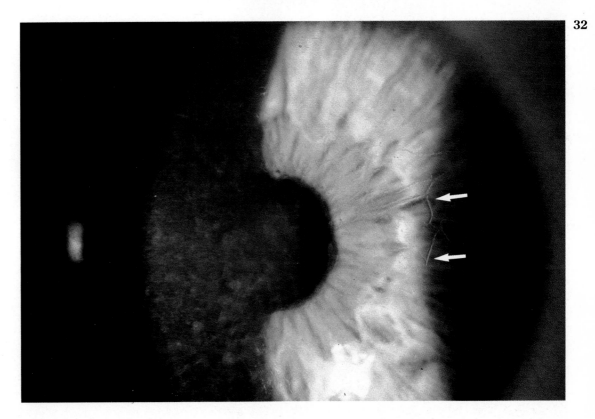

Recurrence of lattice dystrophy

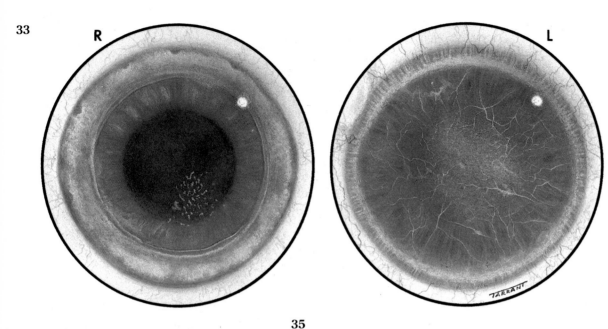

33 The corneas of a 45-year-old man. The left cornea shows advanced lattice dystrophy with central stromal haze. The right cornea demonstrates classic early recurrence of lattice dystrophy five years after keratoplasty. The recurrence has taken the form of multiple, anterior stromal dots, resembling the early signs of the dystrophy.

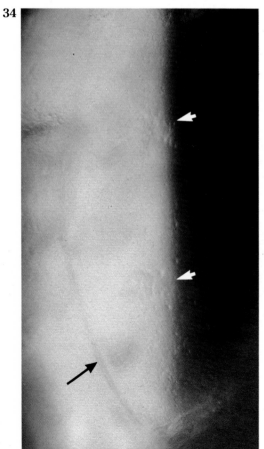

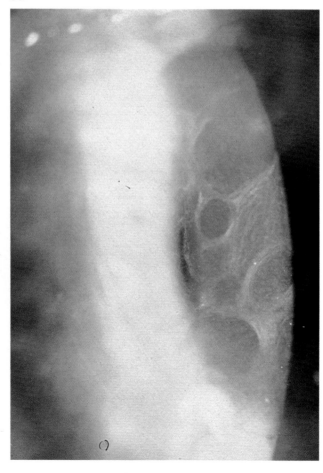

34 & 35 Typical recurrence of the dystrophy (**34**) usually arises near the graft–host junction (black arrow), in the form of refractile, homogeneous dots (white arrows). Atypical recurrence (**35**) can take the form of elevated subepithelial opacities. Light and electron microscopy confirmed the diagnosis of recurrent lattice dystrophy. In the authors' experience, this dystrophy recurs more commonly in the grafts than does granular or macular dystrophy.

Histopathology of lattice dystrophy

36 The histochemical staining of the stromal deposits in lattice dystrophy is very characteristic. The deposits stain orange-red with Congo red, confirming their amyloid nature.

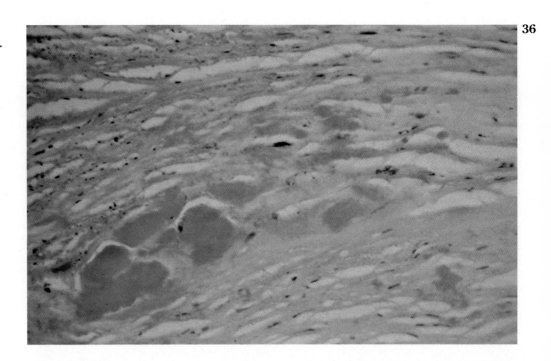

37 When the stained specimen is viewed through a crossed polarising microscope, it manifests green birefringence, which is characteristic of amyloid. Dichroism occurs when the deposits are viewed with polarised light and a green filter.

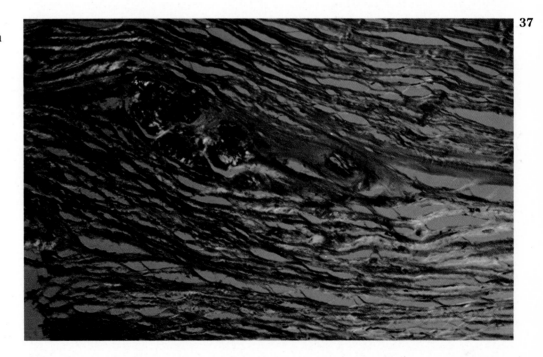

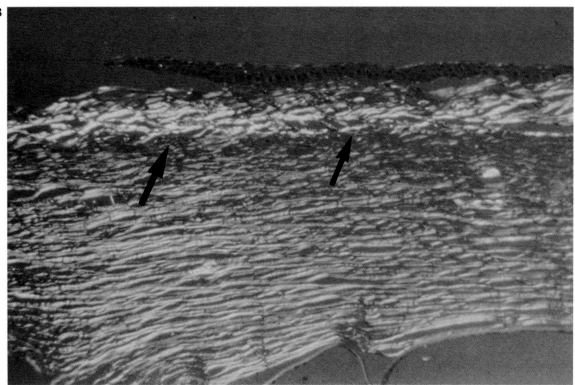

38 In this section, which has been stained for amyloid and then examined by polarised light, increased birefringence of the involved areas is clearly demonstrated. Note that the birefringence is more marked in the superficial stroma (arrows). Electron microscopy of this cornea confirmed that the lesions were amyloid deposits, consisting of extracellular masses of fine, electron-dense fibrils with a diameter of 90 Å. Most of the fibres are highly aligned, which explains the birefringence and the dichroism.

Granular dystrophy (Groenouw I)

Granular dystrophy (Groenouw type I) is an autosomal dominant corneal disorder that has an early onset in the first or second decade of life. Fine, grey-white, discrete dots appear at the central anterior stroma. The intervening stroma remains clear, and vision is not affected in the early stages.

As the dystrophy progresses, the opacities enlarge, coalesce, and increase in number, assuming a variety of shapes resembling breadcrumbs or snowflakes. They gradually spread more peripherally, extending deeper into the stroma. However, the peripheral 2–3 mm of the stroma remain uninvolved, which is an important factor in the differential diagnosis of this disorder from macular dystrophy.

Most patients are either asymptomatic or have only mild photophobia due to scattering of incident light by the opacities. Despite some surface irregularity caused by the involvement of Bowman's layer, recurrent erosions are infrequent.

The substance that accumulates in the stromal lesions is hyaline, a non-collagenous protein containing tyrosine, tryptophan, arginine, and sulphur-containing amino acids; the deposits are produced by abnormal keratocytes in the anterior layers of the stroma.

No treatment is required in most patients, although penetrating keratoplasty may be indicated in those few cases with marked progression of the dystrophy.

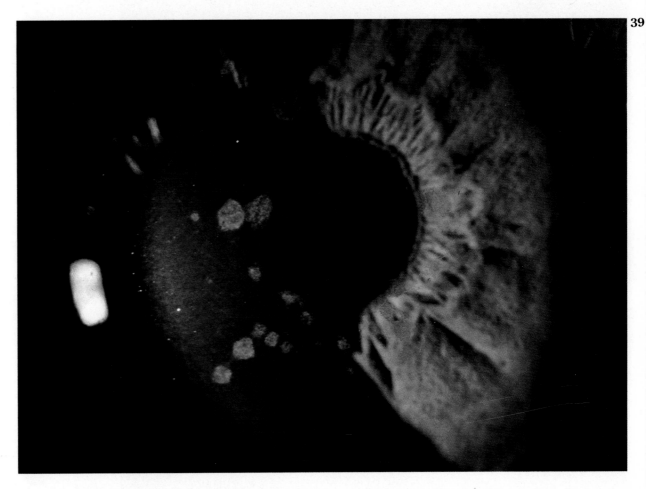

39

39 Granular dystrophy in a 13-year-old girl. The patient was asymptomatic, with no impairment of her visual acuity.

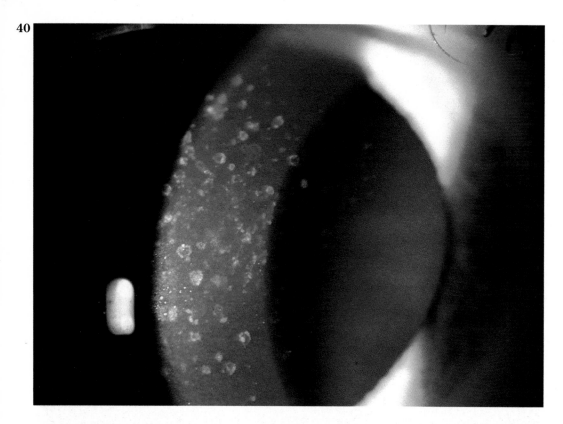

40 The mother of the patient shown in **39** had a similar, but more advanced form of the dystrophy. With oblique focal illumination, the dots, which are situated at the anterior stroma appear opaque, with relatively clear centres.

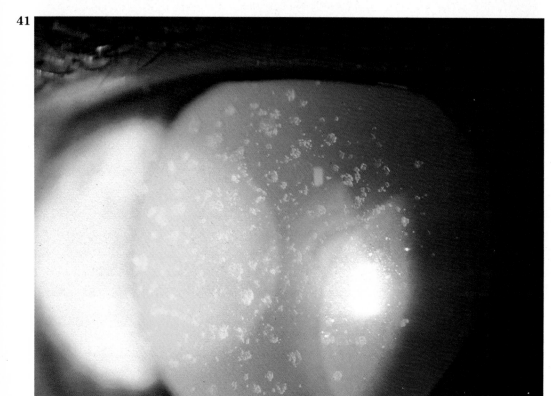

41 On retroillumination, the dots appear to be partially translucent. Some of the families seen in the authors' clinics had a mild variety of the dystrophy, with fewer than 50 granules in a cornea, while other families had a more serious variety with between 50 and several hundred granules. These observations are consistent with other recent reports on granular dystrophy (Moller, 1989).

Progression of granular dystrophy

42 Early granular dystrophy in a 15-year-old boy. Note that the grey-white dots are fine, discrete, and concentrated at the centre of the cornea.

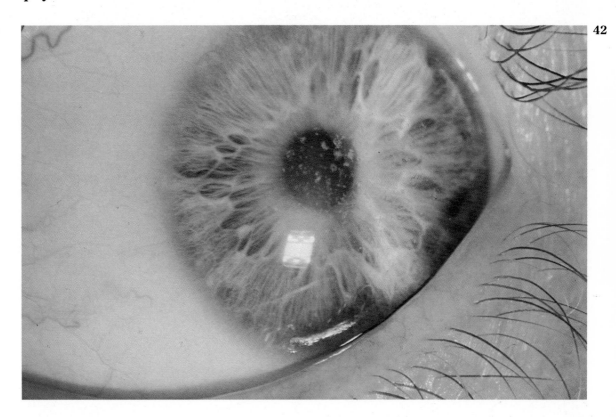

43 A high-magnification photograph of the same cornea shown in **42**. Note that the dots have irregular margins, and that some of them have relatively clear centres. The intervening stroma is clear.

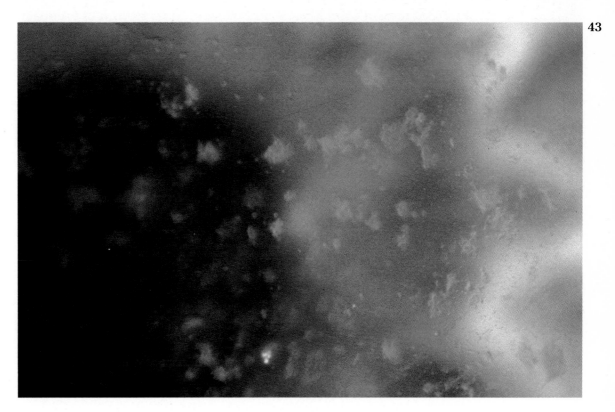

44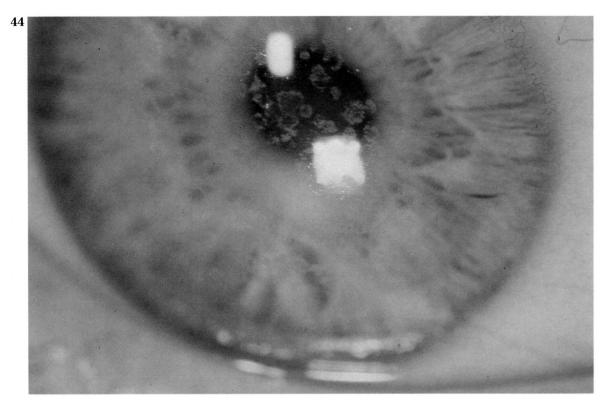

44 & 45 The same patient as shown in **42 & 43**, three years later. The opacities have enlarged and coalesced. High magnification (**45**) reveals that the opacities have assumed a variety of shapes including chains, rings, and snowflakes. The brother of this patient had similar lesions in both corneas. The features of granular dystrophy, especially the presence of erosions and the morphology of the individual lesions, tend to be uniform within families. In those families with few granules the visual prognosis is usually better.

45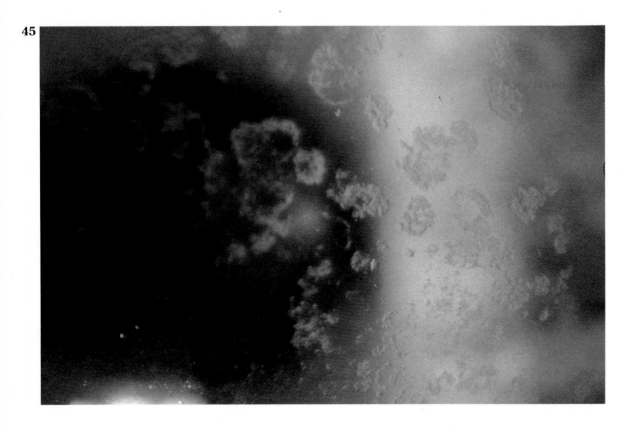

46 Advanced granular dystrophy in a 45-year-old woman. Note that the opacities have coalesced more, with an increase in their size and number. The intervening stroma has become slightly hazy, with a diffuse ground-glass appearance. Penetrating keratoplasty was indicated in this patient because her vision was impaired.

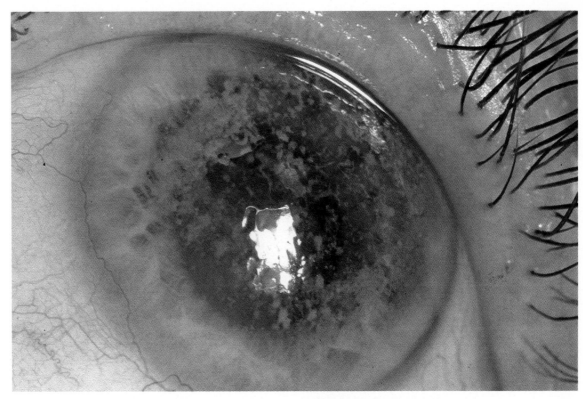

47 The fellow eye of the patient in **46** shows a similarly advanced stage of the dystrophy, with spread of opacities to the corneal periphery. This clinical picture can be confused with macular dystrophy. However, an important factor in the differential diagnosis is that the peripheral 2–3 mm of stroma are not involved in granular dystrophy, as seen in this patient.

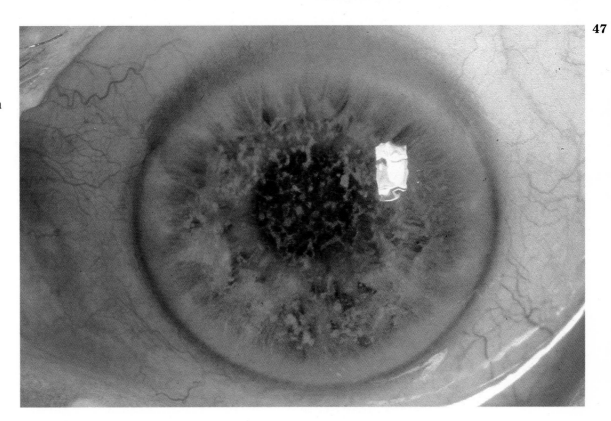

Histopathology of granular dystrophy

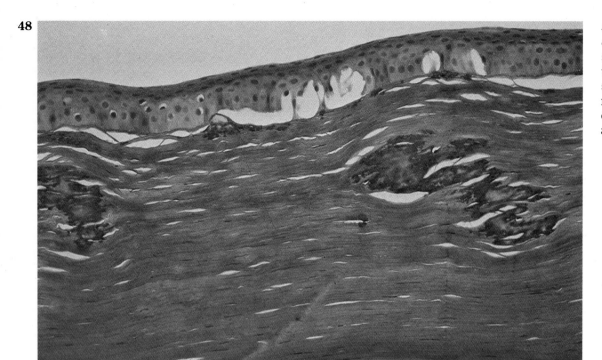

48 Light microscopy demonstrates the characteristic staining of the stromal and subepithelial deposits with Masson's trichrome stain (× 20). Histochemical studies indicate that the deposits are of a noncollagenous protein, hyaline, which contains tryptophan, arginine, tyrosine, and sulphur-containing amino acids.

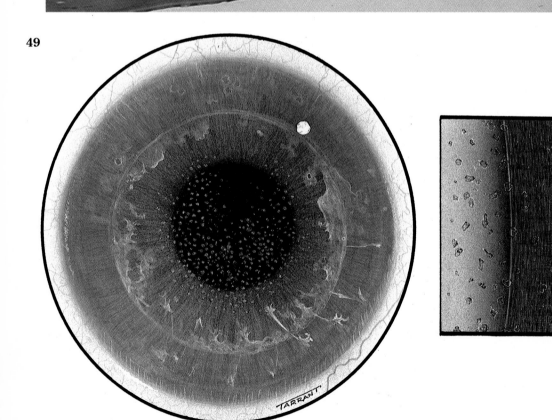

49 Recurrence of the dystrophy following penetrating keratoplasty can be detected as early as 28 months postoperatively, as seen in this patient. Early recurrence has taken the form of very fine, discrete, and partially translucent dots, best seen by retroillumination.

Advanced recurrence of granular dystrophy

50 Preoperative slit-lamp photograph of a 40-year-old patient with granular dystrophy. Visual acuity had been reduced to 6/36, secondary to stromal opacification and corneal surface irregularity. The patient also complained of mild glare due to scattering of the incident light by the stromal opacities.

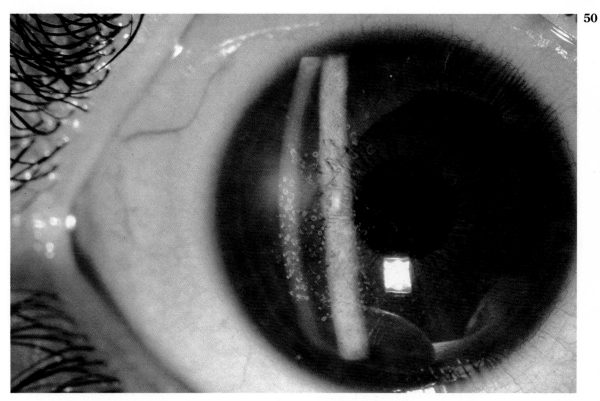

51 Advanced recurrence of granular dystrophy three years after keratoplasty, in the same patient as shown in **50**. Note that the recurrent opacities in the donor cornea have the same shape and distribution as those seen preoperatively.

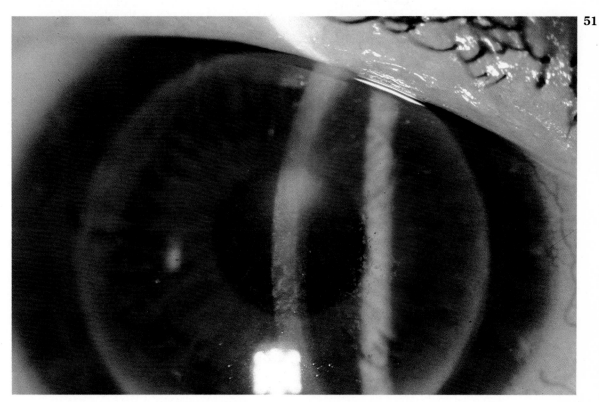

Macular dystrophy (Groenouw II)

Macular dystrophy (Groenouw type II) is the least common of the classic stromal dystrophies (i.e. lattice, granular and macular). Like other recessive disorders, it is more severe and often occurs in pedigrees with consanguineous marriage. The disorder begins in the first decade of life, manifesting as a bilateral, fine, superficial, central corneal stromal haze. Eventually, the entire corneal stroma becomes involved. Multiple, irregular, grey-white nodules develop within the stroma, and surface irregularity occurs with accompanying decreased corneal sensation. However, episodes of recurrent erosions are much less frequent than in lattice dystrophy. Photophobia is a prominent feature, and often seems out of proportion to the clinical involvement. The condition is differentiated from granular dystrophy (Groenouw I) by its recessive inheritance, by the early intervening stromal haze between the multiple opacities, and by the early peripheral involvement that can reach the limbal area.

Macular dystrophy is a genetically determined disorder of the corneal keratocytes, leading to a localised form of acid mucopolysaccharide deposition. Defective catabolic enzymes affect the metabolism of the glycosaminoglycan, causing it to accumulate excessively in the keratocyte. When the keratocyte eventually dies, the glycosaminoglycan is released into the extracellular spaces of the stroma.

Visual impairment by the fourth decade of life may necessitate penetrating keratoplasty. However, the dystrophy may recur in the donor tissue as a result of abnormal glycoprotein production by the affected remaining host keratocytes.

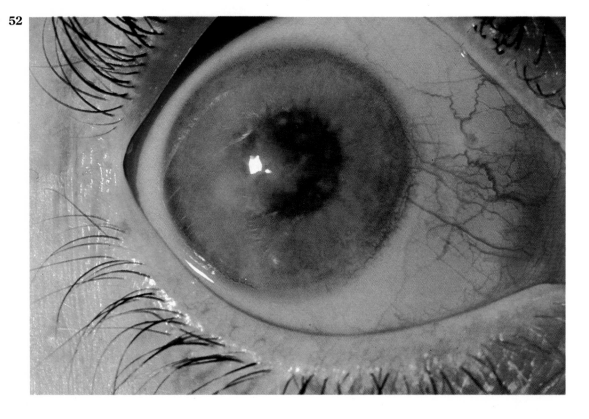

52

52 Classic macular dystrophy in a 45-year-old woman. The presenting symptoms were visual impairment and long-standing photophobia.

Progression of macular dystrophy

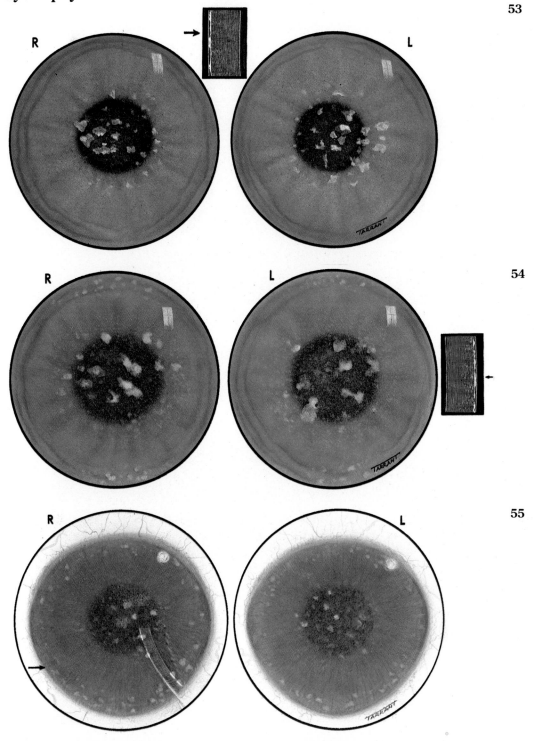

53–55 Follow-up drawings of a patient with macular dystrophy, made over a ten-year period. Note that the early haze in the intervening stroma (**53**) is an important factor in differential diagnosis, as it is not present in patients with early granular dystrophy. **54** shows the patient after three years, and **55** illustrates the degree of progression after ten years.

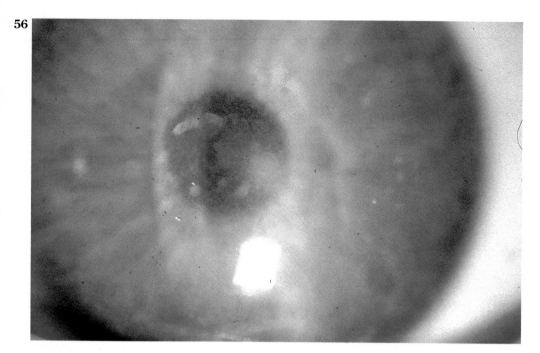

56 Early macular dystrophy starts as a fine, superficial central stromal haze. This progressively spreads to the periphery, developing into multiple nodular opacities that are opaque to oblique focal illumination.

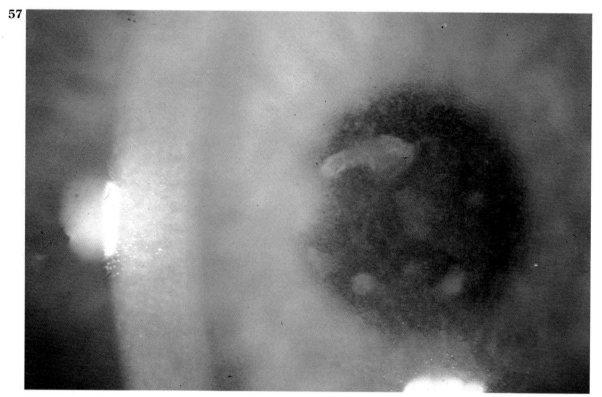

57 Retroillumination highlights the opacities against the background haze. Note that, in contrast with granular dystrophy, the opacities have irregular borders, with hazy surrounding stroma.

58 Early stromal opacities are more superficial and appear initially in the central stroma. As the dystrophy progresses, the opacities involve the entire thickness of the stroma.

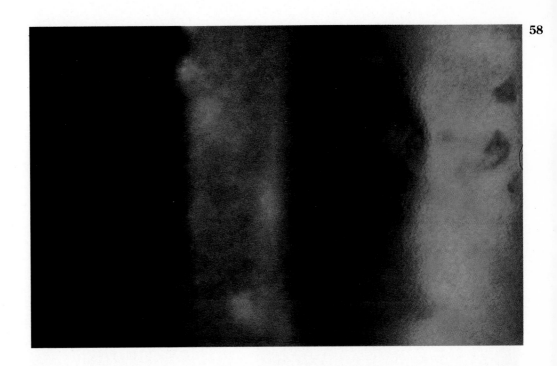

59 In advanced cases the opacities spread to the periphery and can reach the limbus (arrows). This is another important sign differentiating the disorder from granular dystrophy, where the peripheral 2–3 mm of stroma are always spared.

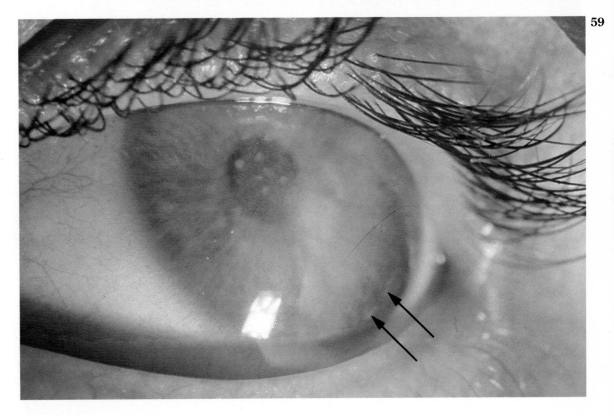

60

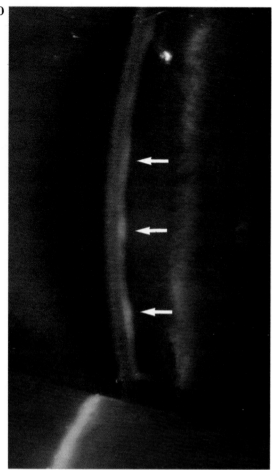

60 The peripheral opacities are more deep and discrete than those in the centre, and may project posteriorly in the anterior chamber (arrows) in advanced cases.

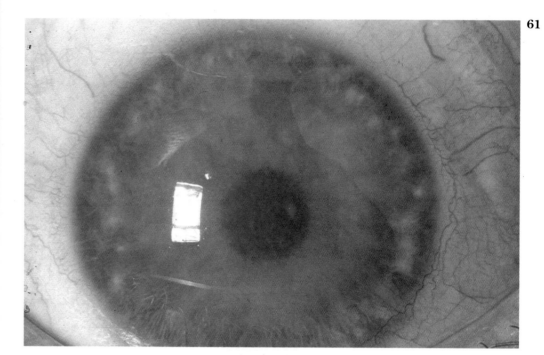

61

61 & 62 Penetrating keratoplasty was indicated in this 35-year-old woman when the advanced dystrophy (**61**) had decreased her best corrected visual acuity to 6/36. Following successful penetrating keratoplasty (**62**), vision improved to 6/6.

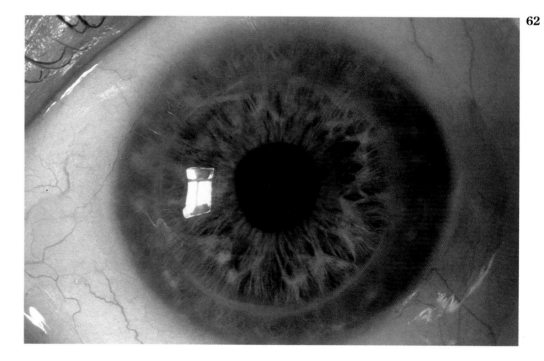

62

Recurrence of macular dystrophy

63 & 64 Macular dystrophy can recur in the donor tissue following penetrating keratoplasty. The recurrence is usually peripheral, and does not impair vision (arrows). The localisation of the recurrence is peripheral because the host keratocytes continue to produce excessive glycoproteins that accumulate and spread to the donor stroma. Most of the recurrences encountered by the authors' patients arose following small grafts (less than 7.5 mm), and were presumably due to the presence of more abnormal host keratocytes in the remaining host stroma.

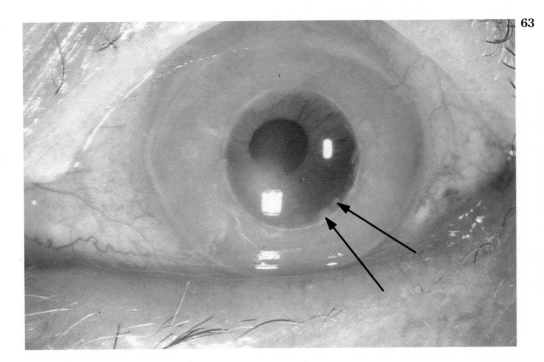

63

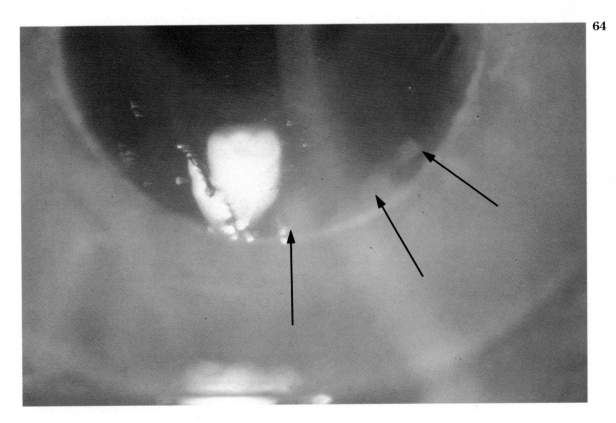

64

Histopathology of macular dystrophy

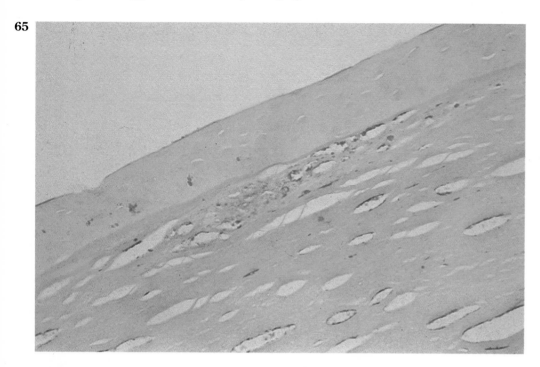

65 & 66 The dystrophy is characterised by the accumulation of glycosaminoglycan within the keratocyte and the surrounding stroma (positive staining with Hale's colloidal iron). Note that the Glycosaminoglycan also accumulates in the sub-epithelial area and Bowman's layer, as well as in Descemet's membrane and the endothelium. Both the intracellular and extracellular glycosamino-glycan accumulations were localised in this cornea by means of silver stains, used in conjunction with electron microscopy. Some of the keratocytes were distended up to three times their normal size by large intracytoplasmic vacuoles.

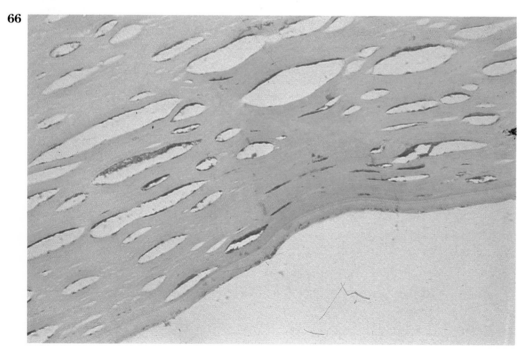

Central cloudy dystrophy (François')

Central cloudy dystrophy was first described by François in 1956. The condition is bilateral, symmetrical, and non-progressive. The inheritance pattern is autosomal dominant. Unilateral cases have also been reported. Although the condition has been noted to occur as early as the first decade of life, it does not progress; both the corneal thickness and the corneal sensation remain intact. Vision is not affected and no treatment is required. The lesions are not macroscopically visible and can only be identified by slit-lamp examination. The central two-thirds of the cornea are involved, with multiple grey opacities in the deep stroma, separated by narrow lines of relatively clear stroma, best seen by broad oblique illumination or scleral scatter.

Central cloudy dystrophy seems clinically identical to the condition termed 'posterior crocodile shagreen of Vogt'. Indeed, it is probably more accurate to use the term 'posterior crocodile shagreen of Vogt' for similar findings, unless multiple family members, especially younger patients, manifest similar changes. Transmission electron microscopy demonstrates a distinctive 'sawtooth' pattern with some of the collagen lamellae located at right angles to others. Interspersed between these areas are patches of abnormal collagen with 100 nm bonding. The uninvolved peripheral and anterior stromal architecture is normal.

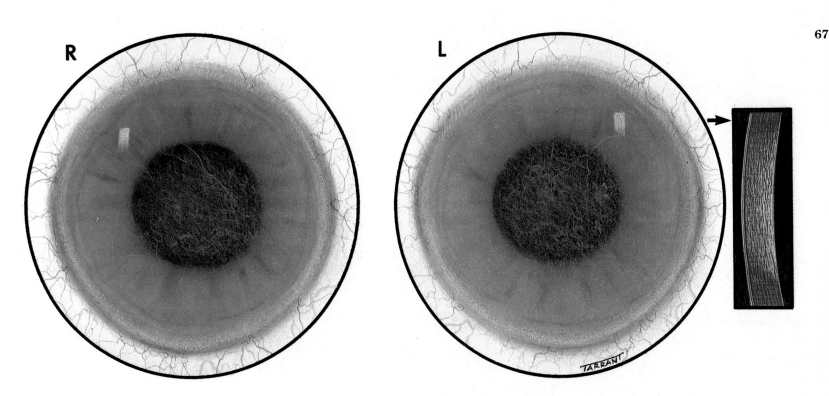

67 Bilateral and symmetrical corneal involvement in a 25-year-old patient with François' dystrophy. Visual acuity is 6/6 in both eyes. The characteristic lesions are not clearly demonstrated by macroscopic examination, and slit-lamp magnification is required to confirm the diagnosis.

68

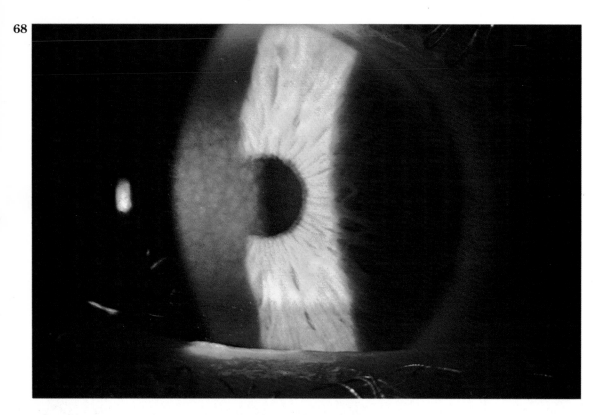

68 Broad oblique slit-lamp examination showing a classic case of François' dystrophy. Multiple greyish opacities involve the central two-thirds of the stroma. These opacities are separated by narrow lines of relatively clear stroma. Note that although the margins of the lesions are fluffy and indistinct, the intervening crack-like areas of clear stroma impart a polygonal structure to the opacities.

69

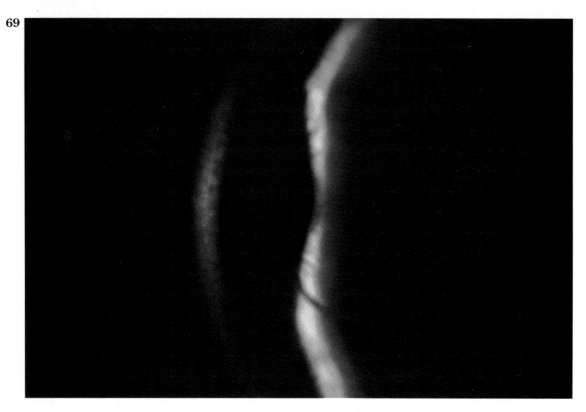

69 A narrow slit-lamp beam shows the deep level of the stromal opacities. Note the normal stromal thickness and the absence of any folds in Descemet's membrane, both of which differentiate this condition from stromal oedema. The diffuse nature of the opacities and their characteristic appearance differentiate them from the discrete lesions of pre-Descemet's dystrophy and cornea farinata.

Central crystalline dystrophy (Schnyder's)

Central crystalline dystrophy is a very rare, bilateral, and symmetrical corneal dystrophy with an autosomal dominant pattern of inheritance. The characteristic corneal lesions were first described by Van Went and Wibaut in 1924, but it was Schnyder who clearly documented the clinical course and the hereditary patterns of this dystrophy. Although the disorder may present unilaterally in a few cases, both eyes eventually become involved in nearly all patients.

The dystrophy usually presents during the first or second decade of life, in the form of minute crystals that involve the central cornea at the level of the anterior stroma. However, the patients remain asymptomatic until later in life, when their vision becomes markedly impaired by the progressive crystalline deposition.

Slit-lamp examination shows a central corneal opacity that has a well-defined border and consists of numerous, fine, polychromatic crystals, best seen with indirect illumination. Although these crystals are initially confined to the anterior stroma, they usually extend to the deep stromal layers as the dystrophy progresses. The cornea retains its normal thickness, with no sign of oedema, as the endothelium does not become involved. A dense corneal arcus is frequently associated with Schnyder's crystalline dystrophy, and may appear early in life.

Light microscopy reveals cholesterol crystals and neutral fats corresponding to the crystalline stromal deposits seen clinically. Bowman's layer is usually involved, with the overlying epithelial basement membrane disrupted by focal aggregations of glycogen. Electron microscopy demonstrates characteristic rectangular spaces that disrupt the normal stromal architecture and represent cholesterol crystals that have been dissolved during processing.

All patients with Schnyder's crystalline dystrophy should be evaluated for systemic lipid abnormalities, as some may have elevated serum cholesterol and triglycerides. However, the association with systemic hyperlipidaemia is not uniform, and it is now believed that this dystrophy represents a localised alteration of cholesterol metabolism in the cornea, which may become modified by systemic hyperlipidaemia.

Differential diagnosis of this dystrophy includes systemic disorders associated with crystalline deposits in the cornea, such as cystinosis, monoclonal gammopathy, multiple myeloma, Waldenström's macroglobulinaemia, and cryoglobulinaemia.

70 Schnyder's crystalline dystrophy in a 45-year-old woman, showing the characteristic numerous, fine, needle-like crystals located in the centre of the cornea. Slit-lamp examination reveals that the crystals are deposited in the anterior stroma and Bowman's layer. The epithelium is normal.

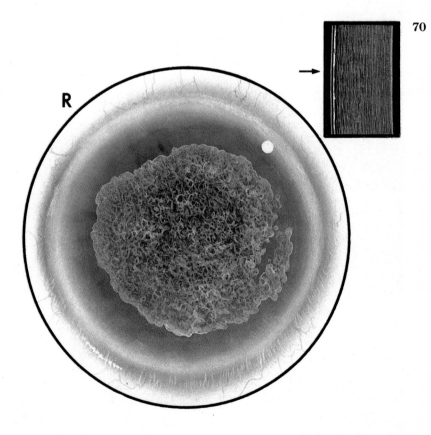

70

71

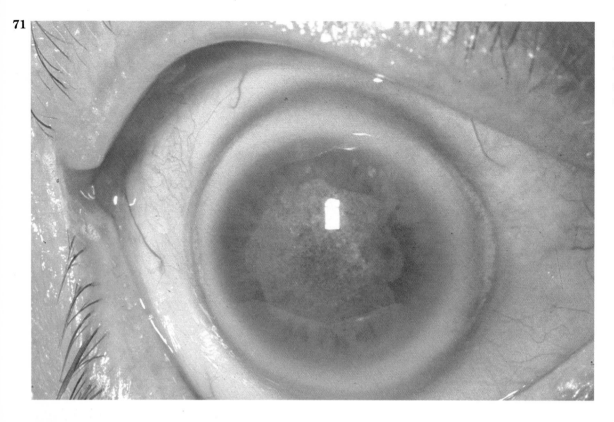

71. Extensive involvement of the central cornea in Schnyder's dystrophy. Visual acuity was reduced to 6/36. Note the dense arcus, a common feature of central crystalline dystrophy, which occurs early in life.

72

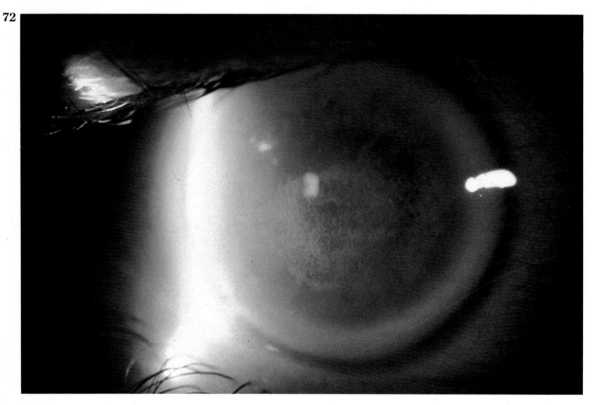

72 Slit-lamp indirect illumination (scleral scatter) reveals the polychromatic nature of the crystals deposited in the anterior stroma. The patient had bilateral and symmetrical stromal lesions. The epithelial surface remains smooth and the corneal sensation is normal.

Progression of Schnyder's dystrophy

73–75 Schnyder's central crystalline dystrophy in three generations of the same family, demonstrating the progressive crystalline deposition. **73** shows the early stage of the dystrophy in a 17-year-old girl. Note the clear intervening stroma between the crystals. In **74** a more advanced dystrophy is seen in the girl's 45-year-old mother. Note the associated corneal arcus. **75** illustrates a very advanced stage of the dystrophy in the 82-year-old grandfather. Note the extension of the crystalline deposits towards the periphery.

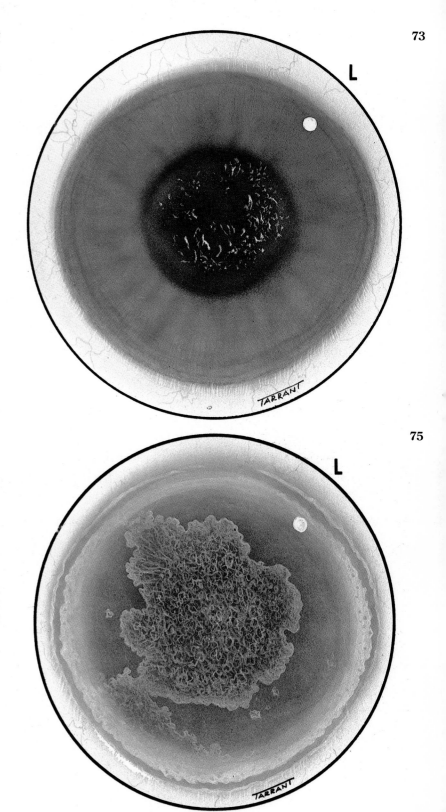

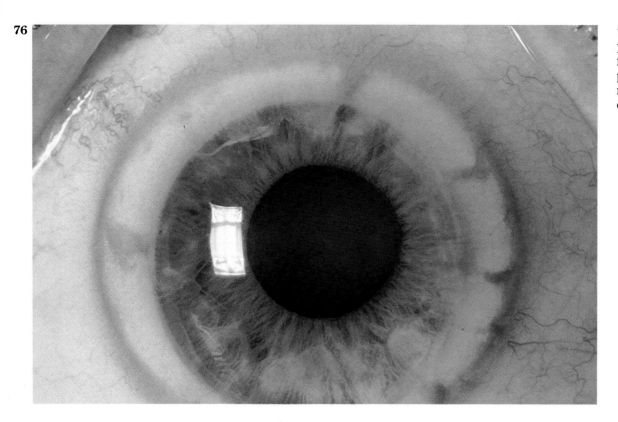

76 A clear corneal transplant three years after penetrating keratoplasty for central crystalline dystrophy. The patient showed no evidence of recurrent crystals in the donor cornea over a ten-year follow-up period.

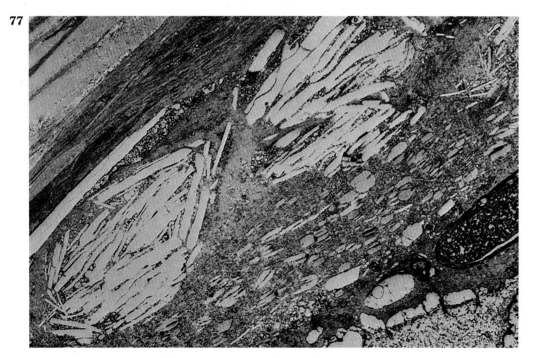

77 Transmission electron micrograph of the stromal lesions in crystalline dystrophy. Note the characteristic oblong and trapezoidal spaces left in the stroma by the cholesterol crystals; the associated disruption of the normal stromal architecture is also visible.

Differential diagnosis

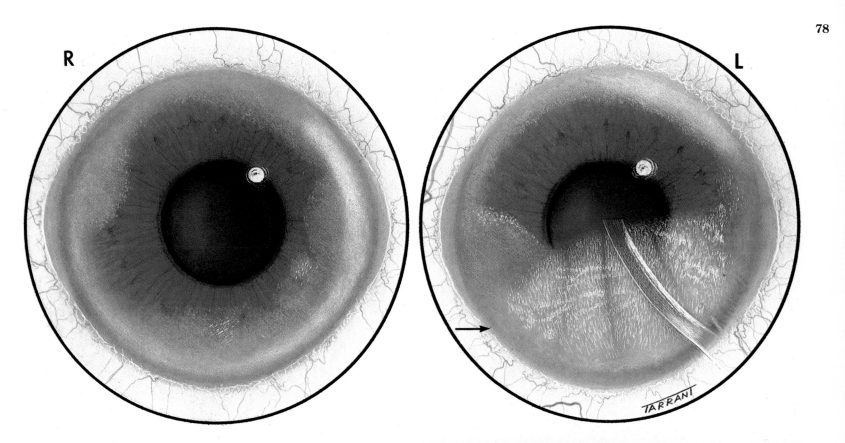

78

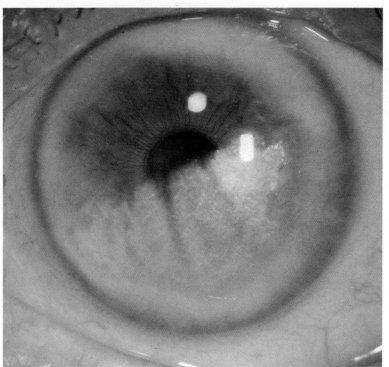

79

78 & 79 Corneal crystalline deposits can be an initial sign of monoclonal gammopathy. The 59-year-old male patient shown in **78** was referred to the authors' corneal clinic, with a provisional diagnosis of Schnyder's dystrophy. Note the atypical arcus formed by the crystalline deposits in both corneas. The left cornea **79** shows a dramatic deep stromal 'Candy-floss' keratopathy, which bears no resemblance to the characteristic central, anterior stromal, crystalline deposits seen in Schnyder's dystrophy. Further investigations confirmed that the patient's corneal crystals were secondary to IgM-kappa chain monoclonal gammopathy.

Pre-Descemet's dystrophies

Pre-Descemet's dystrophies comprise a number of conditions that have been reported with fine opacities limited to the extreme posterior stroma in the pre-Descemet's membrane area. Waring and co-workers (1978) divided these disorders into four clinical types:

- The typical pre-Descemet's dystrophy, which appears between the fourth and seventh decades of life. It manifests in the form of annular, central, or diffuse opacities in the pre-Descemet's area. The condition is bilateral and symmetrical. Differing morphologies of the discrete opacities, including dot-like, comma-shaped, filiform, linear, and stellate shapes, have been described. The inheritance pattern is autosomal dominant.
- Pre-Descemet's dystrophy associated with icthyosis and, occasionally, with pseudoxanthoma elasticum. The grey opacities in the deep stroma have the appearance of snowflakes.
- A polymorphic stromal dystrophy that involves both the mid stroma and the deep stroma, appearing in the form of punctate and filamentous focal grey opacities.
- Cornea farinata, which is an age-related corneal degeneration (*see* p. 84) that presents in the form of pre-Descemet's opacities which are smaller and more polymorphous in appearance than those seen in the typical pre-Descemet's dystrophy.

In all four clinical types, the disorder is asymptomatic and no treatment is required.

Histopathological studies of a case with pre-Descemet's dystrophy demonstrated the accumulation of lipofuscin-like material in the posterior stromal keratocytes (Curran, *et al.*, 1974). This may support the theory that most cases of pre-Descemet's dystrophy represent a degenerative change in the posterior stroma, rather than a true dystrophy.

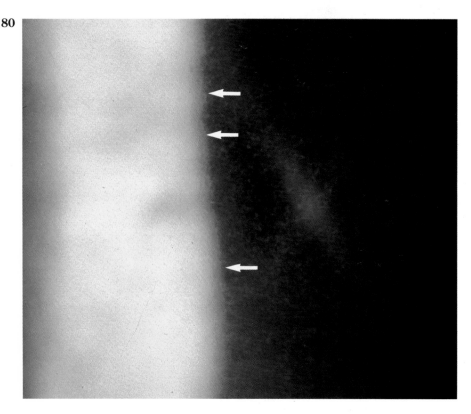

80

80 Slit-lamp photograph of pre-Descemet's dystrophy, demonstrating multiple, subtle, deep stromal, dot-like opacities (arrows). Similar corneal changes were detected in two generations of this patient's family. All the cases were asymptomatic.

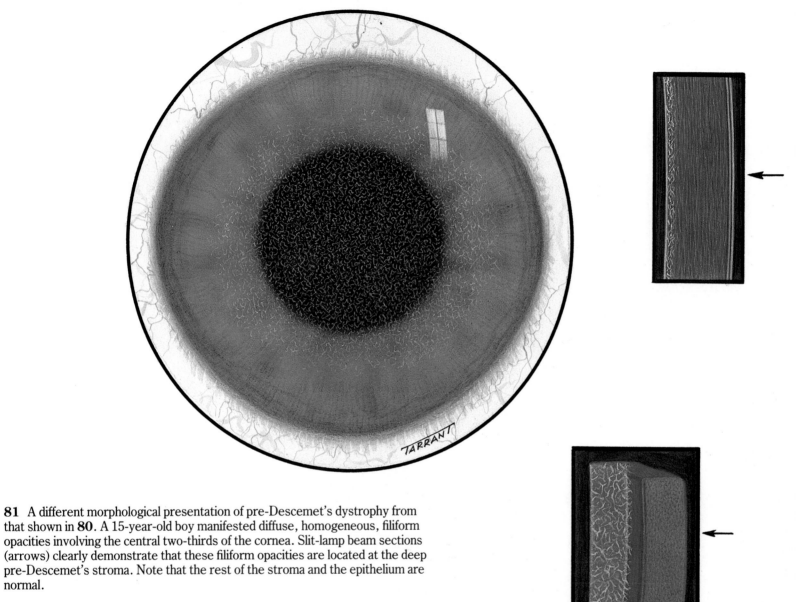

81 A different morphological presentation of pre-Descemet's dystrophy from that shown in **80**. A 15-year-old boy manifested diffuse, homogeneous, filiform opacities involving the central two-thirds of the cornea. Slit-lamp beam sections (arrows) clearly demonstrate that these filiform opacities are located at the deep pre-Descemet's stroma. Note that the rest of the stroma and the epithelium are normal.

3 Endothelial dystrophies

Fuchs' dystrophy

Fuchs' dystrophy is the most common endothelial dystrophy seen in clinical practice. As with some of the other dystrophies, there is considerable overlap between changes that are common in the normal population and early dystrophic alterations that are more rare but ultimately more severe. Fuchs' dystrophy is a bilateral condition, but it is often asymmetrical. Women are affected more severely and three times more frequently than men. Although the disorder often presents after the sixth decade of life, clinical changes may present much earlier in life. The dystrophy shows gradual progression over decades, with three clinical stages: corneal guttata; stromal and epithelial oedema; and corneal scarring.

The inheritance pattern has not been clearly defined, but occasionally it is autosomal dominant. The primary defect occurs in the endothelial cells, and is manifested by the production of a thickened, abnormal collagenous tissue that has the clinical appearance of a thickened Descemet's membrane with multiple discrete excrescences (guttata).

Hypertonic saline drops during the day and hypertonic ointment (sodium chloride 5%) at night may provide symptomatic relief in the early stages of Fuchs' dystrophy with slight epithelial oedema. The pain associated with the rupture of the epithelial bullae can be reduced by the application of a high-water-content bandage soft contact lens. Penetrating keratoplasty is indicated in advanced stages of the dystrophy with marked reduction of visual acuity.

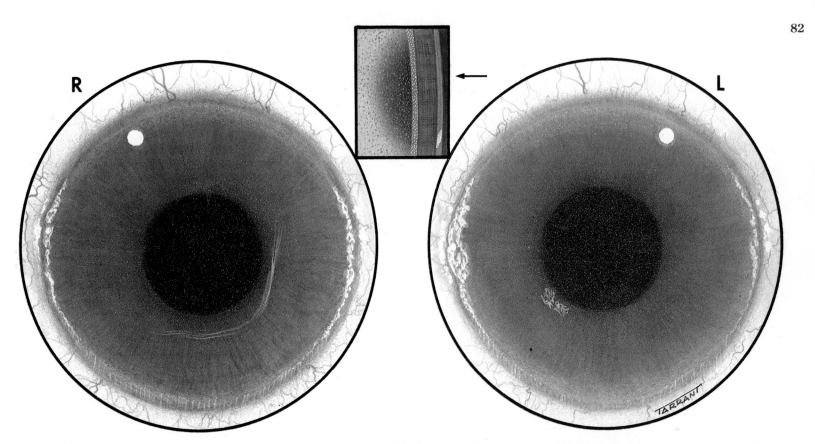

82

82 Stage I: although the patient is asymptomatic in the first stage of Fuchs' dystrophy, pigment dusting and guttata excrescences gradually appear in the posterior cornea.

83

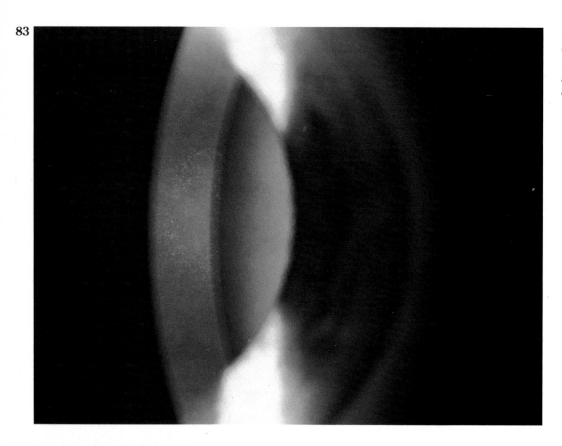

83 Corneal guttata and characteristic pigment dusting of the endothelium are the earliest signs of the dystrophy. Note that the guttata are multiple, central, and not associated with corneal oedema at this early stage.

84

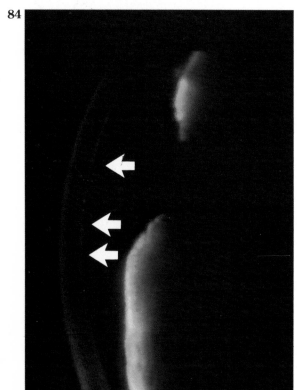

84 Early Fuchs' dystrophy in a 45-year-old woman. A narrow slit-lamp beam reveals the guttata as focal excrescences in Descemet's membrane (arrows).

Progression of Fuchs' dystrophy

85 Specular photomicrograph in an early stage of the dystrophy, demonstrating a few guttata. These appear as dark holes (arrow) in an otherwise normal endothelial mosaic. Best corrected visual acuity was 6/5 and the patient was asymptomatic.

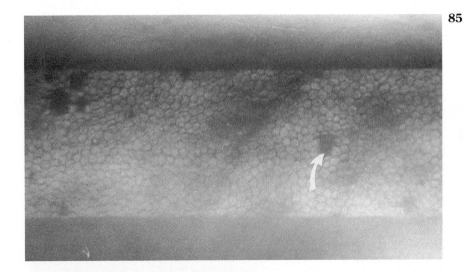

85

86 The same eye as shown in **85**: six months later the guttata (arrow) have become larger, more numerous, and have spread to the periphery.

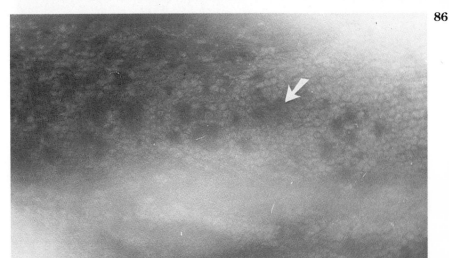

86

87 The same eye as shown in **85 & 86**: eighteen months later the guttata have become very extensive, with marked loss of the endothelial mosaic. Best corrected visual acuity was 6/18. The reduction in acuity was secondary to corneal oedema produced by the failure of the pump function of the endothelial cells.

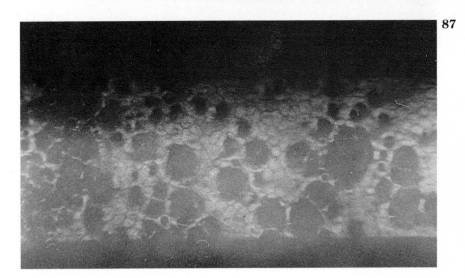

87

88

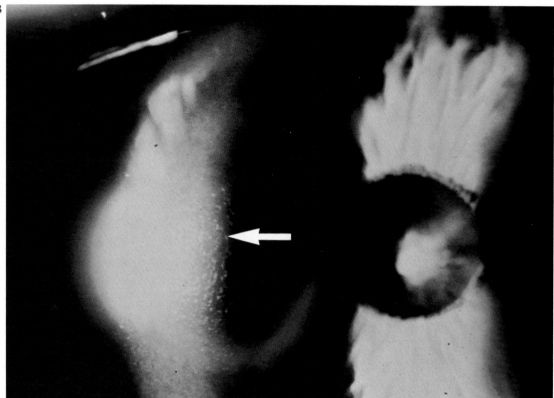

88 The fine, bronze stippling of pigment on the posterior corneal surface (arrow), is often described as having a 'beaten metal' appearance.

89

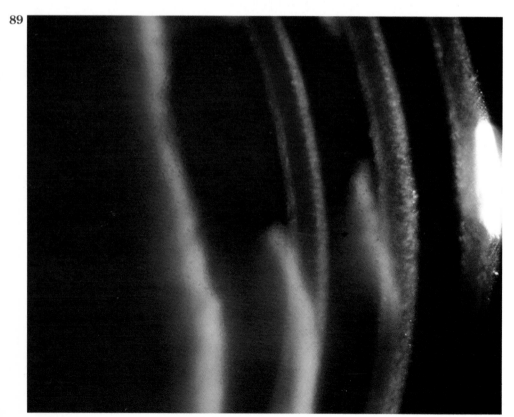

89 Stage II: corneal oedema. In this patient, early stromal oedema is seen in the form of increased thickness of the central corneal stroma, clearly demonstrated by the triple slit-lamp beam. (In healthy eyes the central cornea is normally thinner than that of the periphery.)

90 Epithelial oedema usually develops when the oedematous stroma thickness has increased by about 30%. Note that the early epithelial changes are manifested by slight clouding of the anterior cornea in this patient.

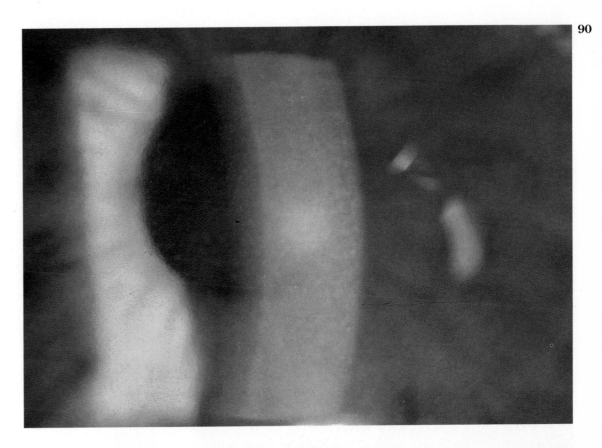

91 As the dystrophy progresses, epithelial microcysts (arrow) start to develop.

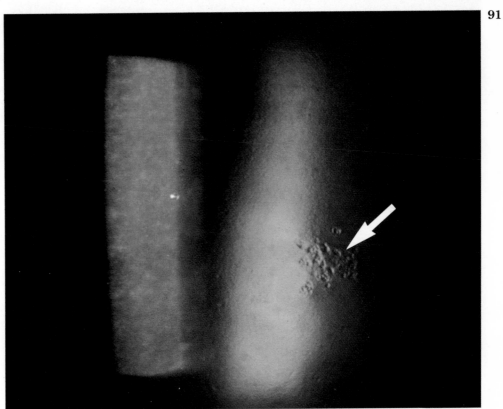

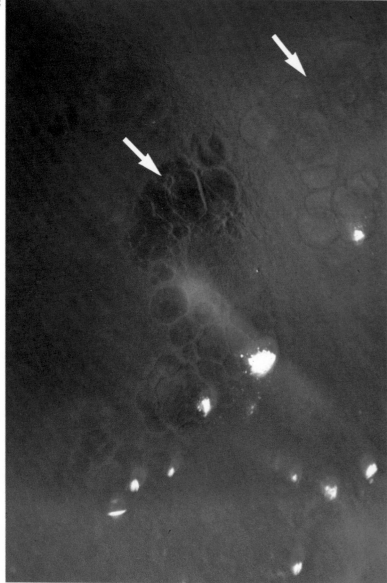

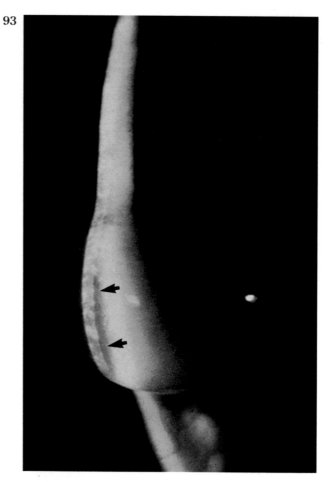

93 A narrow slit-lamp beam clearly demonstrates the coalescent epithelial oedema forming a large bulla (arrows). This is usually followed by epithelial breakdown, which results in severe pain and photophobia. Until visual rehabilitation is achieved by penetrating keratoplasty, a bandage soft contact lens can be beneficial in reducing the discomfort experienced by affected patients.

92 Bullous keratopathy develops because the superficial epithelial cells have tight intercellular junctions, through which fluid cannot pass. The subsequent accumulation of the fluid beneath these barriers leads to the development of epithelial bullae (arrows), best seen by retroillumination.

94 Stage III: subepithelial scarring. With chronic corneal oedema, a diffuse subepithelial sheet of scar tissue separates the stroma from the epithelium. Secondary complications include erosion, ulcers, vascularisation, and decreased corneal sensation.

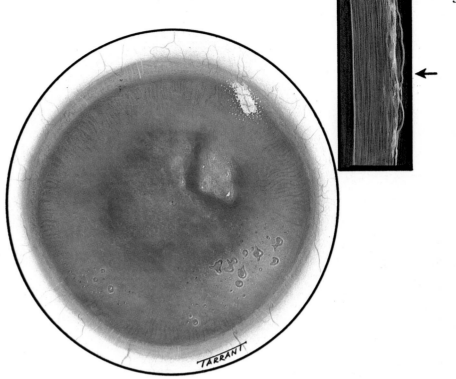

95 An advanced case of Fuchs' dystrophy, with total corneal decompression associated with marked stromal and epithelial oedema. Note the folds in Descemet's membrane, and the irregular light reflex due to surface irregularity caused by epithelial oedema.

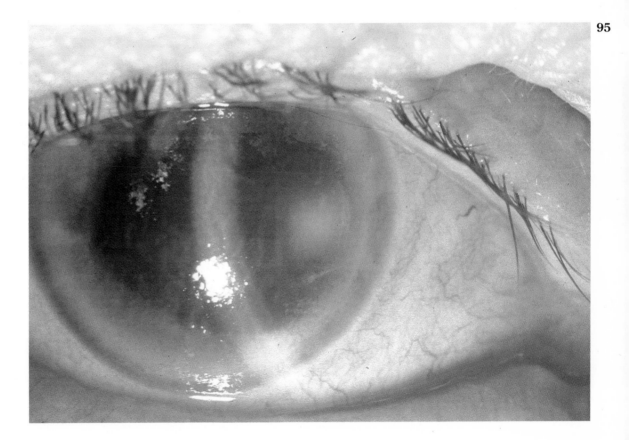

Histopathology of Fuchs' dystrophy

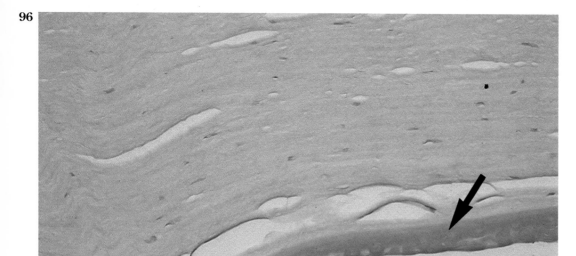

96 Light microscopy demonstrates the thickened Descemet's membrane (black arrow) with its flat-topped excrescences (arrowheads). Endothelial cells located over the guttata are markedly attenuated, and in some places they are even absent (PAS stain × 20).

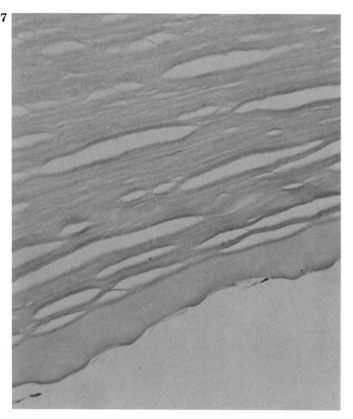

97 High magnification light microscopy clearly demonstrates the excrescences of Descemet's membrane, of which the endothelial lining is so atrophic as to be barely discernible (Van Gieson's stain × 40). When electron microscopy was performed on this specimen it revealed the presence of numerous membrane-bound vacuoles and phagocytised melanin granules in the degenerated endothelial cells.

Posterior polymorphous dystrophy

Posterior polymorphous dystrophy (PPD) is an inherited disorder of the corneal endothelium, characterised by a spectrum of typical changes in the posterior cornea and, less commonly, in the angle and iris structures. Typically, the condition is bilateral, with an autosomal dominant pattern of inheritance. However, PPD may be recessively inherited in some cases, and the authors have seen a few patients with unilateral involvement. A wide variation in expression of the disorder is seen within affected family members.

The age of onset is difficult to determine, as most affected individuals are asymptomatic. However, the fact that corneal oedema and typical vesicles have been noted shortly after the birth of children from families with PPD suggests a congenital onset.

Slit-lamp examination may show a spectrum of findings including vesicles, islands of abnormal endothelium, or a thickened Descemet's membrane. The thickening of Descemet's membrane may be diffuse, in the form of a grey sheet; or localised, giving rise to the characteristic band-like lesions on the posterior corneal surface. In severe cases of PPD, there may be associated corneal oedema. In a minority of affected individuals, fine iridocorneal adhesions may develop as a result of the growth of abnormal endothelium from the cornea, across the trabecular meshwork, and onto the iris. Increased intraocular pressure is found infrequently in patients with PPD. In these cases, especially if there are associated iris changes, the differential diagnosis must include the iridocorneal endothelial (ICE) syndrome.

Severe cases of PPD may require penetrating keratoplasty, with a good visual result in most patients.

98 Posterior polymorphous dystrophy (PPD) in a 25-year-old woman. Note the typical appearance of the vesicles, and their posterior locations. The fellow eye had similar lesions.

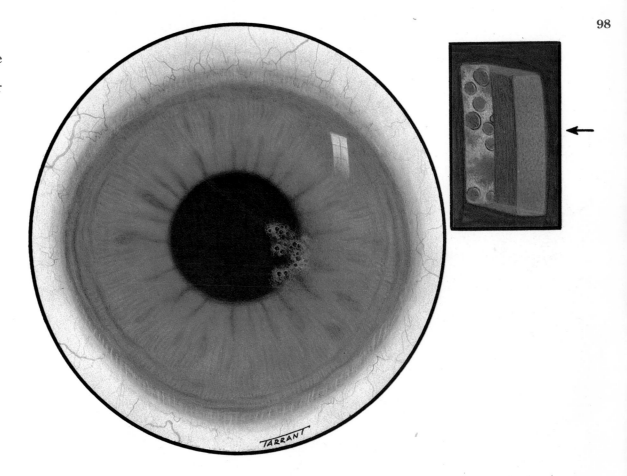

98

99 Isolated, small, posterior corneal vesicles (arrows) in an asymptomatic 19-year-old patient with PPD.

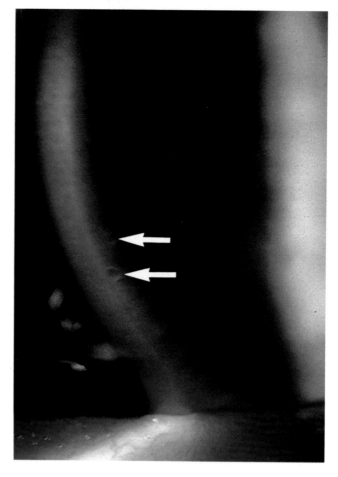

99

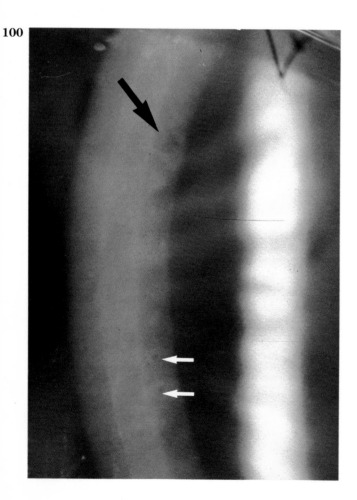

100 The brother of the patient shown in **99**. Note that he has more numerous vesicles, of which some are isolated (white arrows) and some are coalescent (black arrow). Also clearly visible is the thick, sheet-like Descemet's membrane.

101 The father of the two patients shown in **99** & **100** has more severe involvement than his children. Note that the coalescent posterior vesicles have formed larger geographical lesions with dense grey opacification.

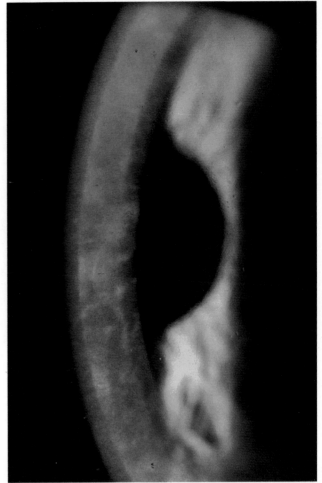

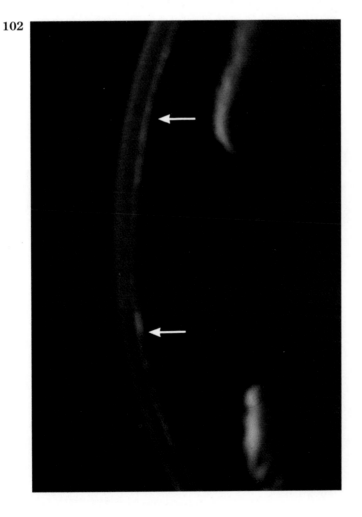

102

102 Thickening of Descemet's membrane is an important sign of PPD, best seen by a narrow optical section (arrows). This thickened membrane consists of a combination of normal anterior Descemet's membrane, abnormal posterior Descemet's membrane, and a collection of posterior collagenous material produced by the endothelial cells.

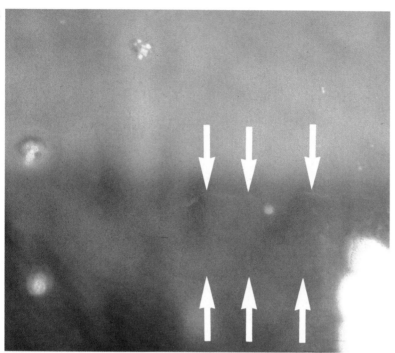

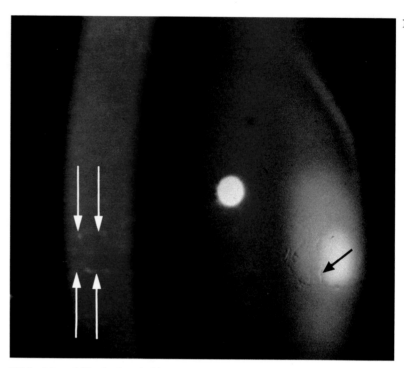

103 Thickening of Descemet's membrane may assume a focal, band-like configuration with a scalloped, irregular margin and non-tapering terminations, as seen in this 45-year-old patient with PPD (arrows).

104 A band-like lesion (white arrows) is more clearly seen in the fellow eye of the patient shown in **103**. Also visible are the typical isolated vesicles, which are highlighted by retroillumination (black arrow).

Progression of PPD

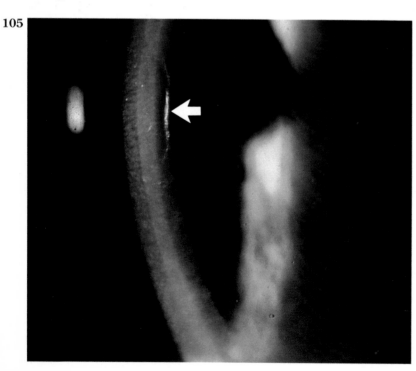

105 Corneal decompensation is not common, as in most cases PPD is non-progressive. Early decompensation is seen here in a 55-year-old patient. Note the stromal thickening, the folds in Descemet's membrane (arrow), and the typical corneal vesicles.

106 Advanced PPD with stromal and epithelial oedema. Note the irregular light reflex. Best corrected visual acuity was 6/36. The patient's father and brother had a milder form of PPD, with no corneal oedema, confirming the wide variation in the expression of the dystrophy among affected members of a given family.

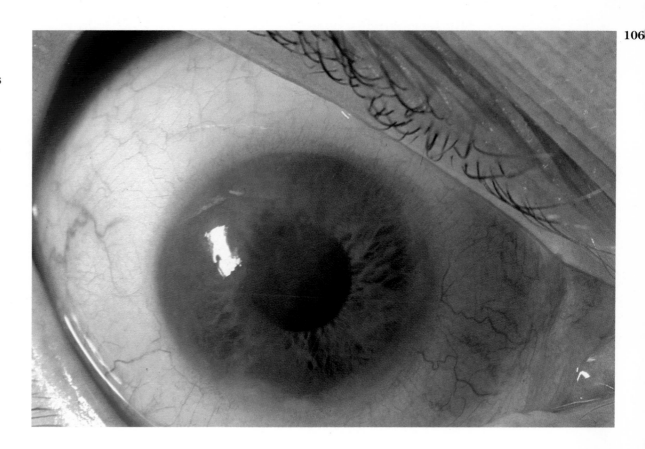

107 Small, localised, basal iridocorneal adhesions (arrow) occur in 10–25% of cases with PPD, as a result of the growth of abnormal endothelium from the cornea, across the trabeculum, and onto the surface of the iris.

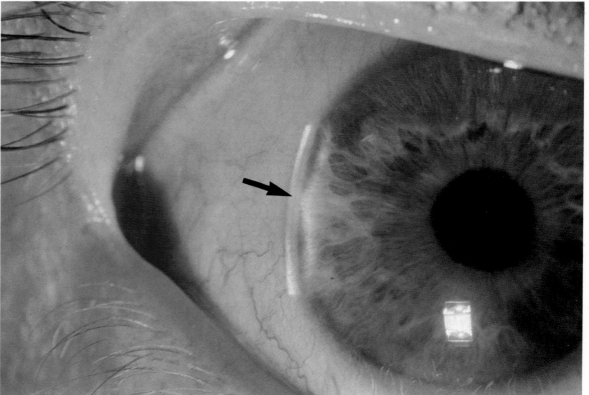

108

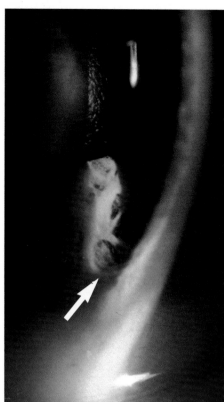

109

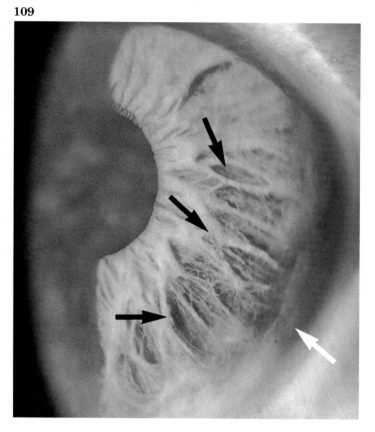

108 & 109 Broad-based iridocorneal adhesions in a case of advanced PPD (white arrows). Broad illumination reveals associated localised stromal atrophy of the iris (**109**) (black arrows), a very rare finding in PPD. The main differential diagnosis of this case is iridocorneal endothelial (ICE) syndrome. Histopathological examination of the corneal button following penetrating keratoplasty confirmed the diagnosis of PPD.

110

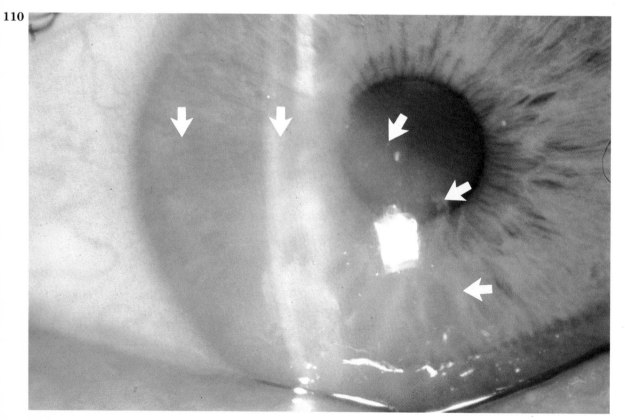

110 Unilateral PPD is another rare presentation of the disorder, and it must be distinguished from the ICE syndrome. This patient presented with localised stromal and epithelial oedema involving the infratemporal quadrant of his right cornea (arrows). Clinical examination and histopathological findings confirmed the diagnosis of PPD. The left eye, however, showed no evidence of the dystrophy, both clinically and by specular microscopy.

111 Calcific band keratopathy, seen here in a 25-year-old patient, is a rare association of PPD. The patient's 60-year-old father also had bilateral PPD, but had never developed band keratopathy, confirming the variation of expression of the disorder among affected members of the same family.

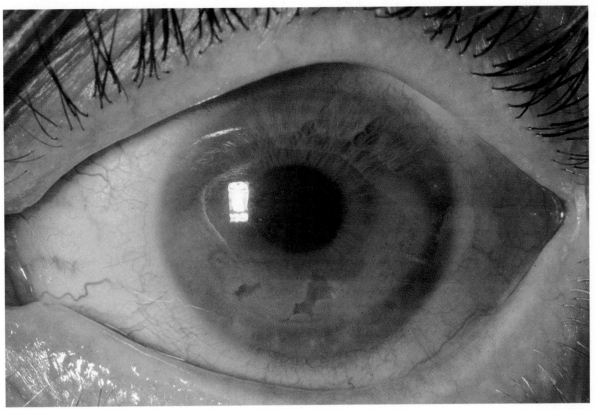

112 Specular microscopy of a case of PPD, showing abnormal dark areas in the endothelial mosaic (arrows). These areas represent islands of abnormal endothelium.

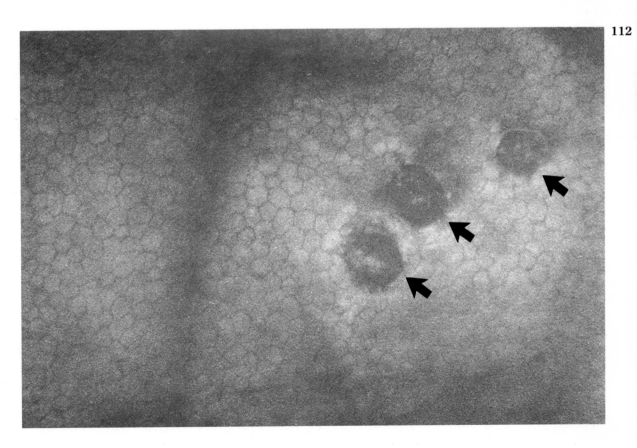

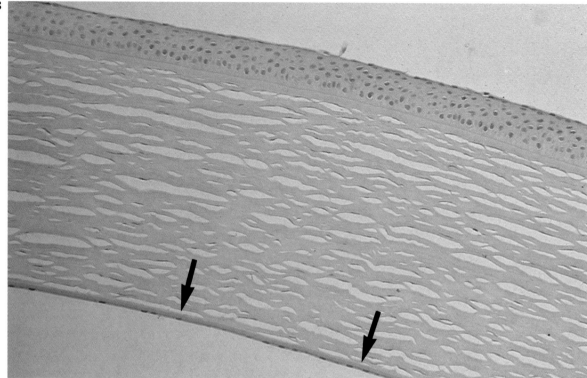

113 Histopathological specimen from an advanced case of PPD. Note the thickening of Descemet's membrane (arrows). Transmission electron microscopy of the endothelium showed abnormal, epithelial-like cells with prominent microvilli, occurring in multiple layers. Immunofluorescent staining of PPD endothelium with antikeratin antiserum demonstrated fluorescence corresponding to the area of epithelial-like cells.

Congenital hereditary endothelial dystrophy

Congenital hereditary endothelial dystrophy (CHED) is the most common congenital dystrophy seen in clinical practice. It has two distinct modes of inheritance. The autosomal recessive type tends to be more severe, presents with corneal clouding at birth, remains nonprogressive in most cases, and may be accompanied by nystagmus. In pedigrees with an autosomal dominant pattern, corneal clouding appears later and is often preceded by irritation and photophobia. The opacification is slowly progressive in some of these cases, and nystagmus is less frequently seen.

In CHED, affected corneas demonstrate a diffuse, marked stromal thickening, giving the cornea a ground-glass appearance that varies from a mild haze to a more confluent. milky opacification. Slit-lamp examination reveals bilateral epithelial and stromal oedema involving the entire cornea. Small, more dense, white stromal opacities and diffuse grey thickening of Descemet's membrane may be present. Intraocular pressure is normal and corneal sensation remains intact.

The basic problem in CHED seems to be one of defective formation of the endothelium *in utero*. Histopathological examination shows profound stromal oedema, attenuation or absence of the endothelium, and changes in the posterior structure of Descemet's membrane.

The success of penetrating keratoplasty in CHED is limited in many cases by the presence of amblyopia. However, good results have been reported when grafting has been performed in the first few months after birth.

114 Diffuse stromal and epithelial oedema in a patient with congenital hereditary endothelial dystrophy (CHED). The cornea has a typical ground-glass appearance.

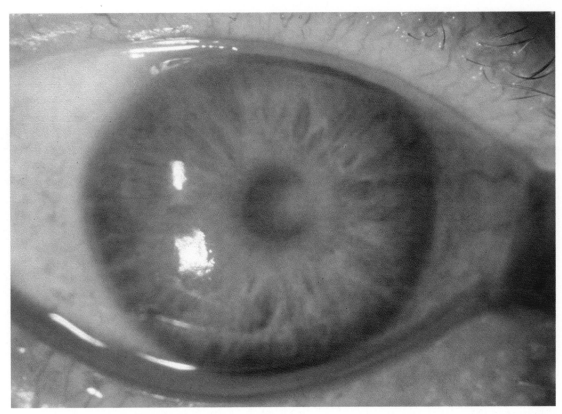

115 Broad optical section of the same patient as shown in **114**. Note that the diffuse increase in stromal thickness has given the cornea a uniformly diffuse, milky appearance.

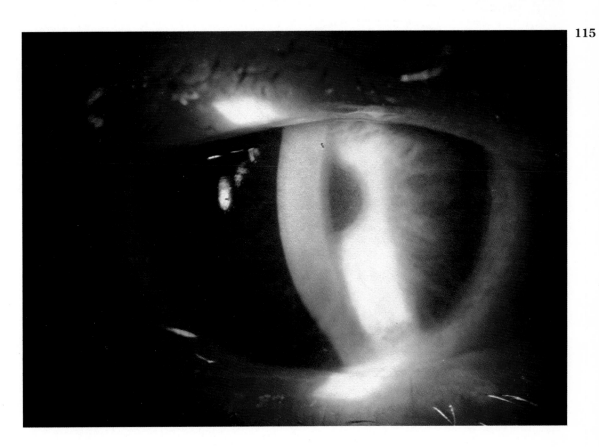

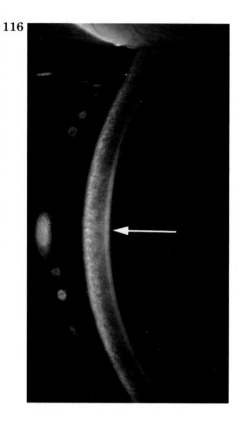

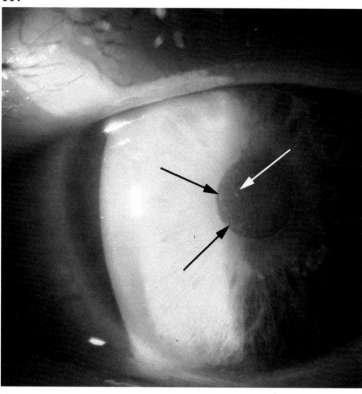

116 A narrow slit-lamp beam reveals the associated thickening of Descemet's membrane (arrow). Following penetrating keratoplasty, histological examination of this cornea revealed increased collagen fibril diameter, an irregular Descemet's membrane, and severe endothelial abnormalities.

117 Indirect illumination reveals the presence of discrete, white dots in the stroma (arrows).

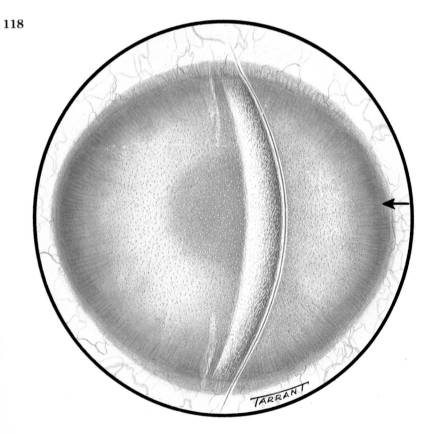

118 Autosomal recessive CHED in a 10-year-old girl. Note that the corneal involvement is more severe than that in the autosomal dominant case seen in **114** & **115**. The marked stromal thickening has given the cornea a more diffuse, milky appearance.

4 Keratoconus

Keratoconus is a non-inflammatory axial ectasia of the cornea, with an estimated incidence of 1 in 20,000. The condition has a slowly progressive course in most cases, and results in high degrees of irregular, myopic astigmatism. Progression is most likely to occur in patients aged between 10 and 20 years, decreasing slightly between 20 and 30, and much less likely after 30. The disorder affects all races. Although earlier studies suggested a female preponderance, other reports, including a study that the authors have published recently, showed males to be predominantly affected (68%). Both eyes are affected in 85% of cases, although there may be asymmetrical severity of involvement.

In keratoconus the progressive corneal thinning leads to a localised conical protrusion of the cornea. The cone may be round or oval, and is located near the visual axis or inferior to it. There may be apical thinning of the cornea to half of its normal thickness. Fine, apical, linear, anterior stromal scars appear in many cases, representing the repair of breaks in Bowman's layer.

Other characteristic slit-lamp signs are also found in keratoconus patients. Vogt's striae are vertical lines, running parallel to the steep axis of the cone, that represent folds in the deep stroma and Descemet's membrane. The visibility of the corneal nerves is usually increased, and the base of the cone may be partially or completely encircled by an epithelial ring of the iron pigment ferritin (Fleischer's ring). Ruptures in Descemet's membrane may occur in advanced cases, causing acute stromal oedema referred to as acute hydrops. The oedema usually resolves in 3–4 months, leaving a residual scar.

In early cases the cone may not be easily discernible and a high degree of suspicion is required to make the diagnosis. Keratoscopy may be required to confirm the diagnosis, and should be performed in any adolescent with progressive myopic astigmatism. The pathogenesis of keratoconus is still unknown. The absence of family history in 95% of cases suggests that the corneal changes represent an ectatic corneal degeneration, not a true dystrophy. Electron microscopy studies indicate that the earliest changes may occur in the basal cells of the epithelium. These cells degenerate, releasing proteolytic enzymes that destroy the underlying tissues. Degenerative changes in the keratocytes near the cone have also been detected.

Many ocular and systemic conditions have been associated with keratoconus including vernal catarrh, retinitis pigmentosa, contact lens wear, Down's syndrome, Marfan's syndrome, osteogenesis imperfecta, atopic dermatitis, and Ehlers–Danlos syndrome.

Keratoconus patients are managed with hard contact lenses when spectacles become inefficient. Penetrating keratoplasty is indicated when contact lenses no longer correct the irregular astigmatism, when there is contact lens intolerance, or when the axial cornea is permanently scarred. In a recently published study, the authors have reported that 93% of the grafts performed for keratoconus patients remained clear over a follow-up period of six years, and that 81% achieved a final corrected visual acuity of 6/12 or better (Sharif and Casey, 1991).

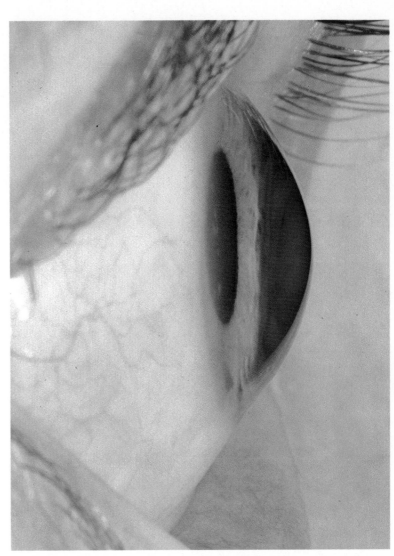

119

119 Lateral view of the cornea, illustrating the characteristic conical profile of a patient with keratoconus. This sign is produced by the marked central corneal ectasia.

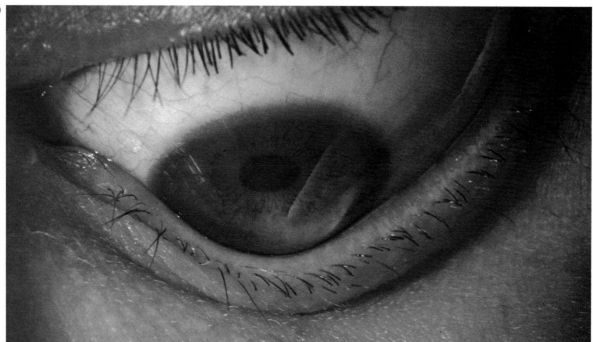

120 Munson's sign. Note the V-shaped indentation of the lower lid, produced by the ectatic cone on downgaze.

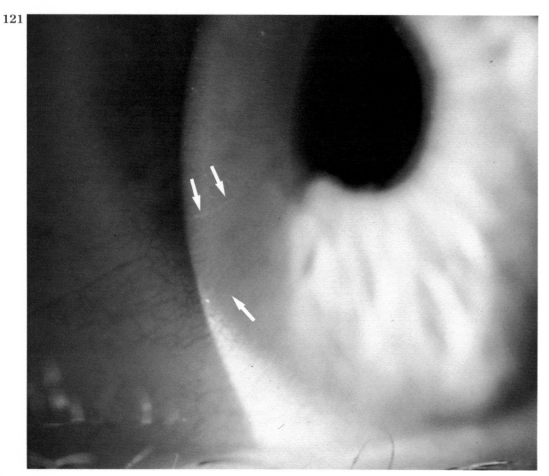

121 Broad oblique slit-lamp illumination commonly reveals large corneal nerves (arrows), the visibility of which usually increases in keratoconus patients.

122 Fleischer's ring is an epithelial pigment ring that partially or completely encircles the base of the cone in keratoconus. Formed by the deposition of ferritin in the basal layer of the epithelium, it is another important slit-lamp finding, and occurs in most cases of the disorder. In this patient the incomplete Fleischer's ring (arrows) demonstrates that the cone is oval, and infratemporal in location.

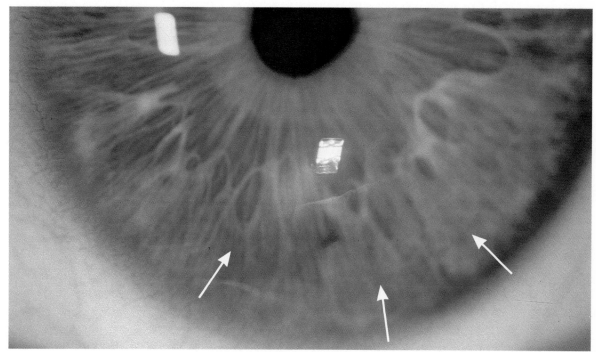

123 A rounded and more central cone than that seen in **122**. The borders of the Fleischer's ring (arrows) are darker and more visible when viewed with cobalt-blue illumination. Note the associated apical scarring.

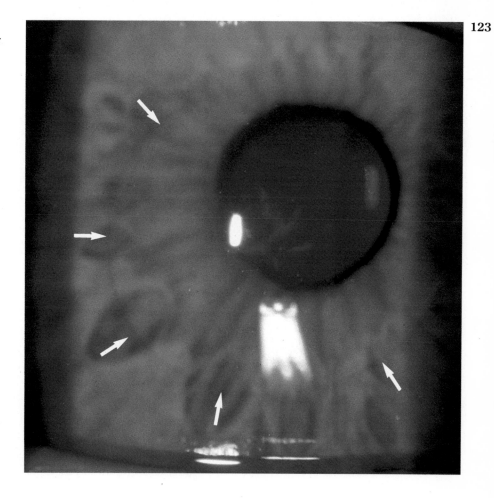

124

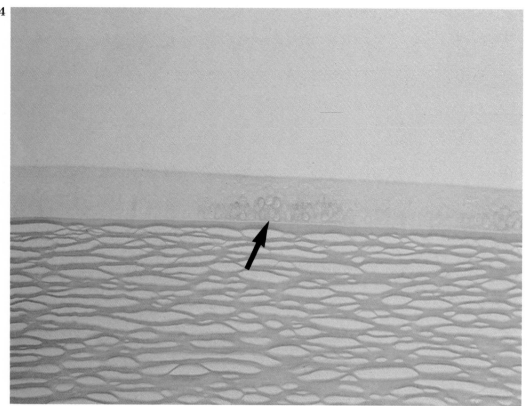

124 Histopathology of Fleischer's ring. Perls' staining of the corneal button of a keratoconus patient demonstrates that the iron pigment is deposited in the basal layers of the epithelium (arrow).

125

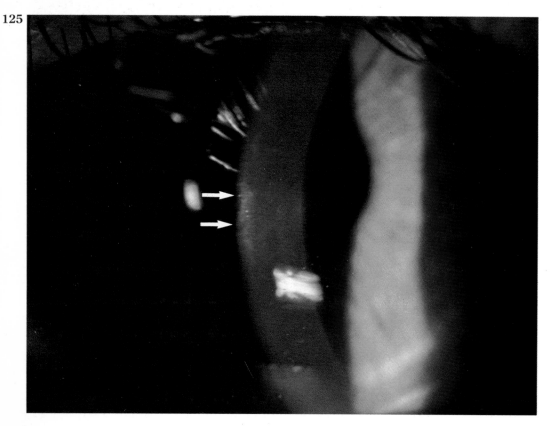

125 Apical scarring commonly occurs in patients with keratoconus. The fine, linear, anterior stromal scars (arrows) result from the repair of breaks in Bowman's layer at the apex of the cone.

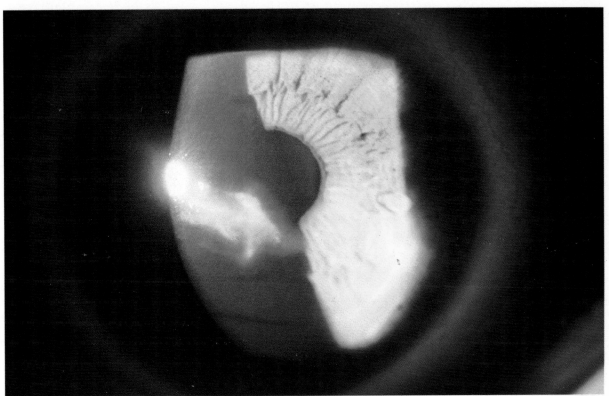

126 & 127 The more dense and deeper stromal scarring seen in some cases of keratoconus is evidence of a previous attack of acute hydrops. This patient had encountered a hydrops attack two years previously, which resolved, leaving a dense scar (**126**). The narrow double slit-lamp beam (**127**) demonstrates the deep stromal location of the scarring (arrows).

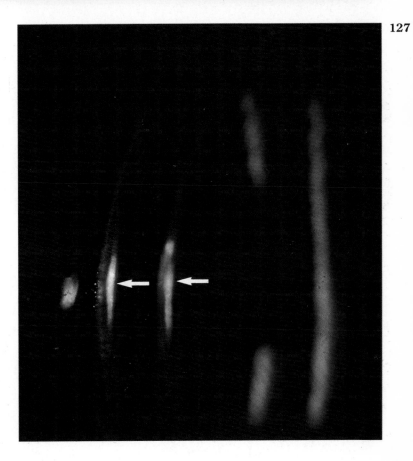

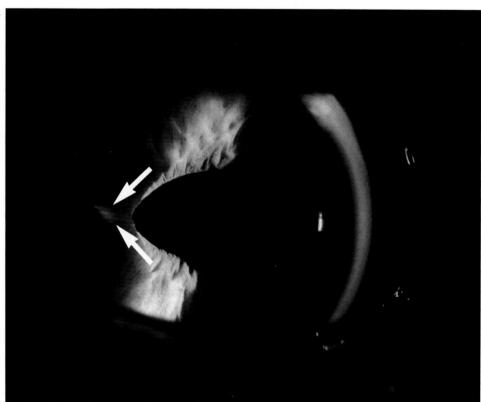

128 Rezutti's sign is a sharply focused beam of light (arrows) near the nasal limbus, produced in some keratoconus patients by lateral illumination of the cornea. The beam is central to the limbus in moderate cases, and more peripheral as the cone progresses.

129

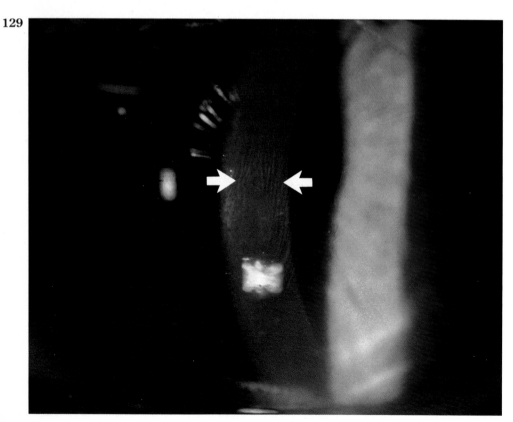

129 Vogt's striae (arrows) are fine, vertical folds that are seen at the level of Descemet's membrane and the deep stroma. They run parallel to the steep axis of the cone.

130 & 131 When external digital pressure is applied to the globe, Vogt's striae temporarily disappear. These high-magnification slit-lamp photographs illustrate Vogt's striae before (**130**) and after (**131**) digital pressure. Their transient disappearance is evidence that they are of a mechanical, rather than a pathological, nature.

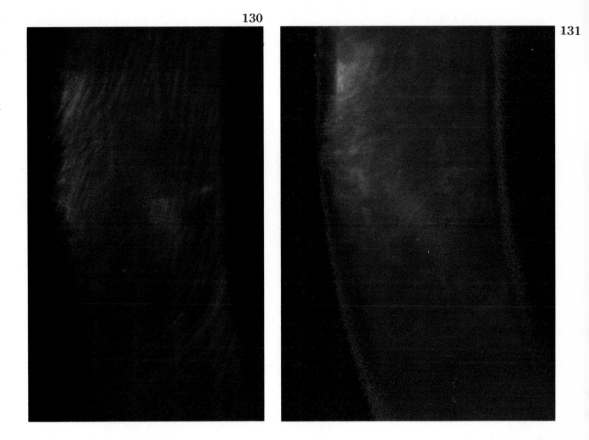

132 Tears in Descemet's membrane can occur in advanced cases of keratoconus, leading to acute localised stromal oedema in the area of the cone (acute hydrops). The oedema resolves in 3–4 months, leaving a residual scar. This picture was taken three weeks after an attack of acute hydrops.

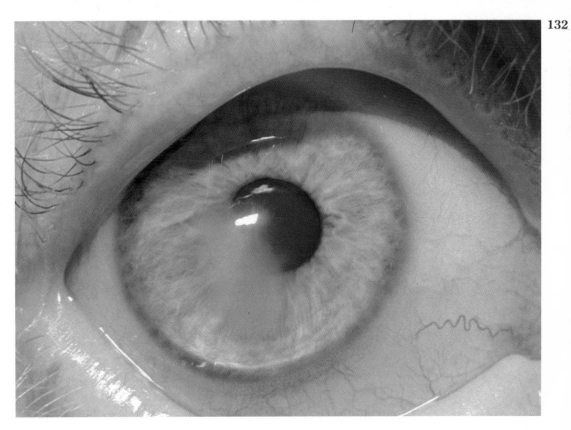

133

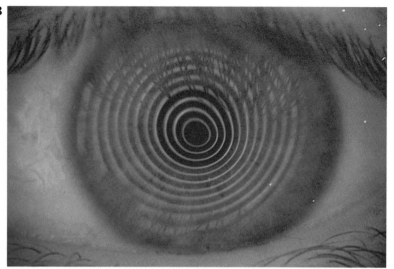

133 Early diagnosis prior to the appearance of the previously mentioned slit-lamp signs can be achieved by keratoscopy. Keratoconus was suspected in this 17-year-old patient with progressive myopic astigmatism; keratoscopy revealed a characteristically ovoid central mire, caused by infratemporal steepening of the cornea.

134 Computer-assisted analysis of photokeratoscopic images has recently been used to provide a more detailed evaluation of the shape of the anterior corneal surface. The colour-coded topographic maps generated using these methods allow inspection of the contour from the central to the peripheral cornea, and can be useful for detecting early corneal irregularity in suspected keratoconus patients.

134

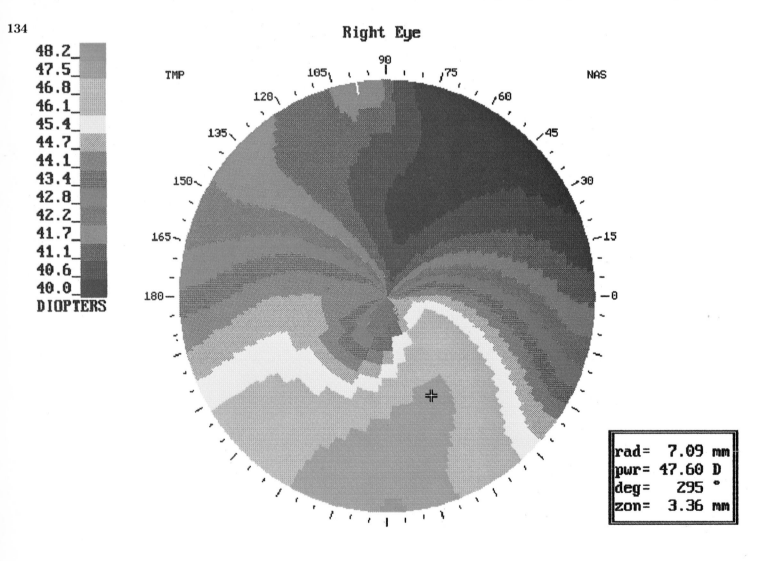

Associated conditions

135 Vernal keratoconjunctivitis is occasionally associated with keratoconus, as seen in this patient. Note the giant papillae at the superior tarsal conjunctiva, with their typical flat-topped 'cobblestone' appearance. The associated yellowish white mucous discharge has a characteristic ropy consistency (arrows). It is postulated that chronic eye rubbing is the main cause of the development of keratoconus in vernal patients.

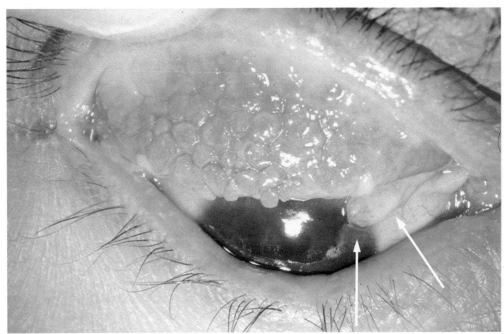

135

136 Cataract in a 25-year-old atopic patient with advanced keratoconus. Note the marked thinning of the central cornea, highlighted by the narrow slit-beam (arrows). A triple procedure (extracapsular cataract extraction, intraocular lens implantation, and penetrating keratoplasty) was required for the visual rehabilitation of this patient.

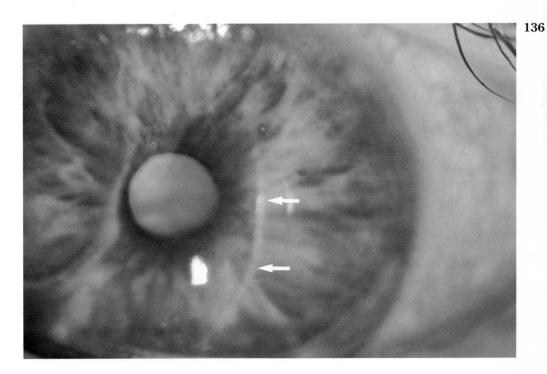

136

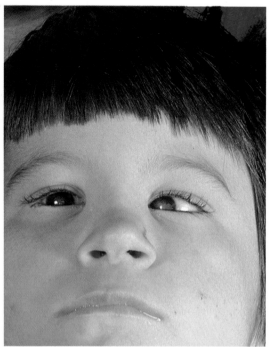

137 & 138 Keratoconus is reported to occur in up to 8% of patients with Down's syndrome. Acute hydrops is more frequently encountered in these patients than the rest of the keratoconus population. This 7-year-old girl presented with acute hydrops of the left eye. Note the epicanthal folds and the left esotropia.

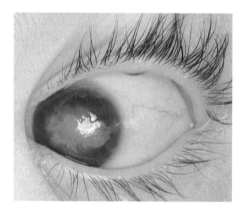

138

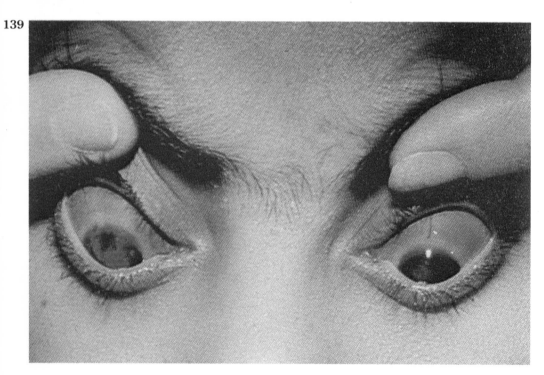

139 Osteogenesis imperfecta congenita is associated with bilateral keratoconus in this patient. Note the blue sclera and the presence of Munson's sign.

5 Age-related corneal degeneration

Some degenerative corneal lesions are considered to be normal ageing processes. In most cases the patients are asymptomatic, with no impairment of vision. Age-related conditions include:

- White limbal girdle of Vogt.

- Corneal arcus (arcus senilis).
- Cornea farinata.
- Corneal guttata.
- Crocodile shagreen of Vogt.

White limbal girdle of Vogt

140 White limbal girdle of Vogt is a degenerative corneal change directly associated with age. It is present in 55% of the population aged between 40 and 60 years, while in patients over the age of 70 the incidence increases to more than 90%. It occurs in the form of a narrow, crescentic, chalky white subepithelial line in the nasal and/or temporal limbal areas of the cornea within the interpalpebral fissure, with no clear zone between it and the limbus. It is best seen with combined retroillumination and scleral scatter (arrows). Histologically, the lesion represents a degeneration of the subepithelial collagen, which is probably related to exposure to sunlight.

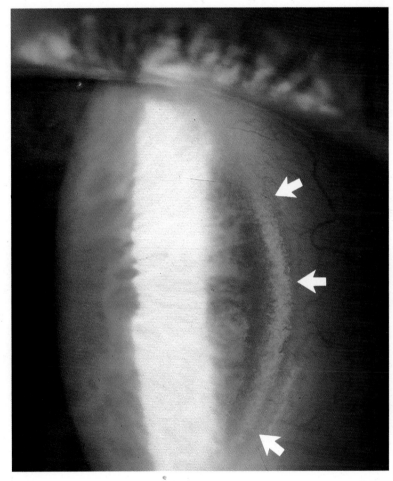

140

Corneal arcus (arcus senilis)

Corneal arcus is the most common age-related corneal degeneration. It occurs in 60% of the normal population aged between 40 and 60 years, and in almost all people over the age of 80. Races of African origin are affected at an earlier age than whites, and the condition tends to occur ten years later in women than in men.

Arcus is a band of yellowish white deposits that initially occurs in the inferior aspects of the peripheral limbus. It then develops in the superior aspects, eventually encircling the entire corneal circumference. It is always separated from the limbus by a clear interval of cornea that is 0.2–0.3 mm in width.

The formation of the arcus is related to the increasing permeability of the limbal vessels with age, which allows low-density lipoproteins to pass into the cornea. The presence of corneal arcus in a young patient (i.e. less than 40 years of age) is an indication that the plasma lipid levels should be checked. The most common association is with type II and III hyperlipoproteinaemias, and it has been shown that the presence of arcus in young patients is a significant risk factor for coronary heart disease.

141

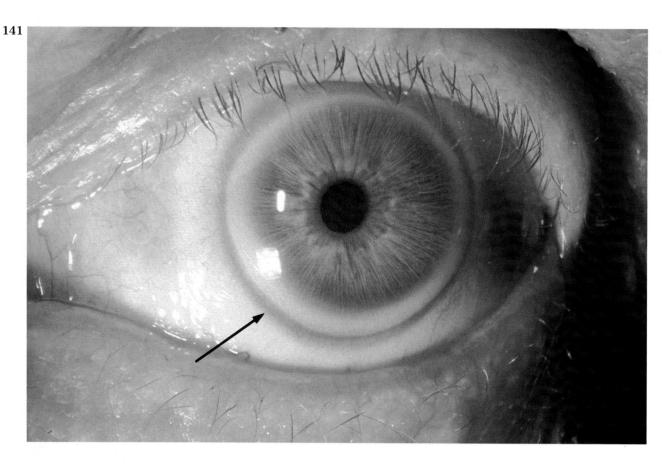

141 Arcus senilis in a 65-year-old man. Note the clear zone separating the arcus from the limbus (arrow).

142 High-magnification slit-lamp photograph of the patient shown in **141**. Note that the arcus has a sharp, well-demarcated peripheral border (black arrow), separated from the limbus by a clear interval, and a diffuse central border (white arrow).

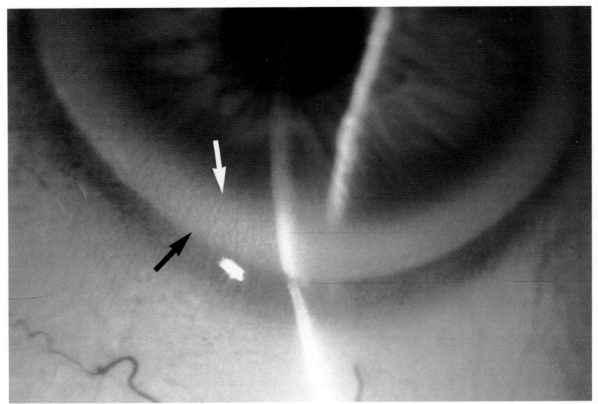

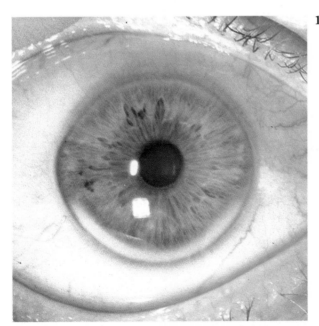

143

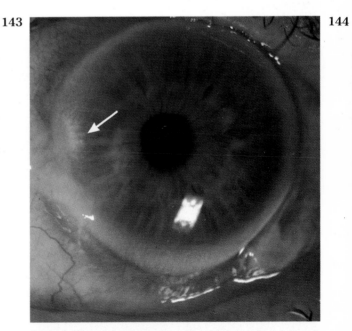

144

143 Early corneal arcus in a 45-year-old woman. Note the characteristic early distribution of the deposits: the inferior periphery is more markedly involved than the superior, and the interpalpebral area has not yet been involved.

144 A 70-year-old woman with a history of peripheral corneal inflammation (at 9 o'clock) that has lead to a denser arcus formation at that site. Note the localised central deviation of the arcus (arrow).

Cornea farinata

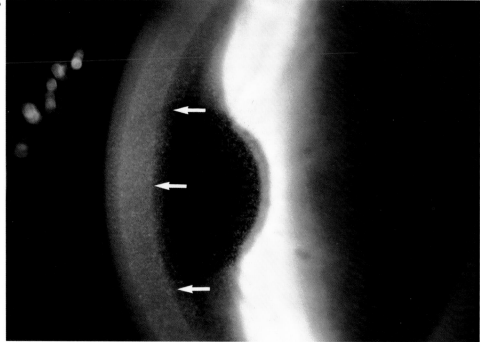

145 Cornea farinata is an age-related degeneration that occurs in the form of very fine, discrete, dust-like opacities scattered throughout the deep stroma, giving it a floury appearance (arrows). The condition is usually bilateral, although some unilateral cases have been reported. Histological studies have shown vesicles in the posterior keratocytes that contain lipofuscin (a degenerative pigment that accumulates in old cells). The affected patient is totally asymptomatic as these opacities cause no visual impairment. The opacities of cornea farinata bear a marked resemblance to the lesions found in pre-Descemet's dystrophies (*see* **80**), although they are smaller and are usually seen at a later age.

Corneal guttata

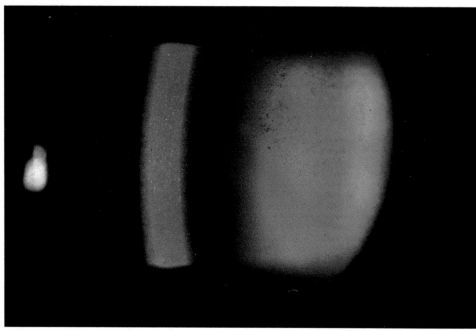

146 More than 70% of the normal population over the age of 40 years have one or more corneal guttata. These lesions represent changes in Descemet's membrane as its posterior, non-banded portion progressively thickens with age. Localised nodular thickening arises, disturbing the regular mosaic of the endothelial cells. Corneal guttata are products of abnormal endothelial cells; they do not cause endothelial decompensation in most cases. In some patients the guttata develop at the periphery of the cornea at an early age (20–30 years), in which case they are called Hassall–Henle bodies.

Crocodile shagreen of Vogt

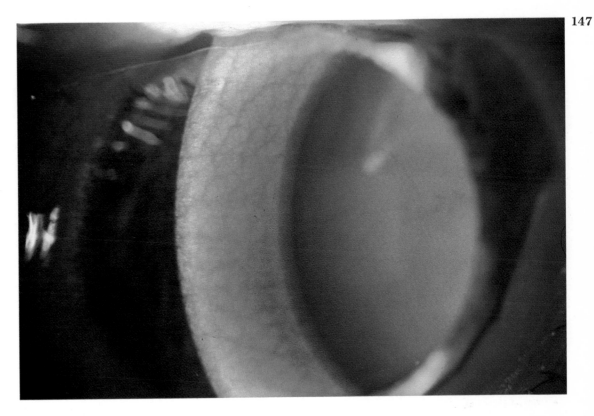

147 & 148 Crocodile shagreen of Vogt is a degenerative corneal condition that presents as greyish white, polygonal stromal opacities separated by relatively clear spaces (**147**). Often a bilateral condition, it affects the central portion of the cornea. In most cases the corneal changes are located in the anterior third of the stroma (anterior crocodile shagreen), although in some cases they can occur posteriorly (posterior crocodile shagreen). The latter presentation has a clinical appearance similar to that of François' central cloudy dystrophy (*see* **68**). As the corneal thickness remains normal (**148**), patients are usually asymptomatic; visual acuity is rarely reduced. The mosaic appearance is related to the arrangement of the anterior stromal lamellae that enter Bowman's layer obliquely. In conditions associated with relaxation of the normal tension on Bowman's layer, for example, prolonged hypotomy and ageing, ridges form, indenting the epithelium to produce the mosaic pattern.

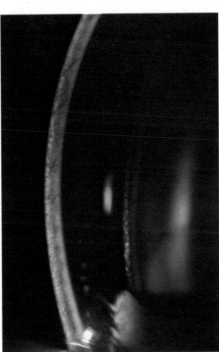

6 Calcific corneal degeneration

Corneal calcification is traditionally divided into two distinct types:

- Calcific band keratopathy.
- Calcareous degeneration.

Calcific band keratopathy

The classic form of corneal calcification seen in clinical practice is band keratopathy. Typically, the calcium deposits are extracellular, occurring in Bowman's layer, in the basement membrane of the corneal epithelium, and in the superficial stromal lamellae. Band keratopathy can appear as a degenerative change following chronic ocular disease, repeated ocular trauma, or systemic disease with elevated serum calcium or phosphate. The most common cause of band keratopathy in children is chronic uveitis, especially in association with juvenile rheumatoid arthritis. Band keratopathy has also been associated with the prolonged use of pilocarpine drops, which contain phenylmercuric nitrate, a preservative that has been shown to be responsible for the gradual deposition of calcium salts in the cornea.

Band keratopathy can rarely occur in the primary type in patients with no ocular or systemic disease. The calcific band develops within the palpebral fissure and is separated from the limbus by a clear zone. The band begins in the corneal periphery and extends towards the centre from both sides, affecting the central area last. There are numerous holes within the band, where corneal nerve endings penetrate Bowman's layer.

The reasons for this process of calcium deposition in the classic band shape are not clearly understood, but it is known that calcium and phosphate are present in blood and interstitial fluids at levels exceeding those at which they are soluble. Precipitation can therefore be triggered by pH elevation, evaporation of tears, or an increase in the concentration of either calcium or phosphate. The evaporation of water, with the subsequent concentration of calcium salts, favours precipitation of the calcium within the palpebral fissure. Initially, the deposition of calcium may be limited to the anterior layers, where there is an accumulation of lactic acid; calcium precipitation occurs to a lesser degree, or is absent, in the deep stroma, as the pH there is lower. There is also no deposition at the limbus (the clear zone), where the buffering capacity of the blood prevents a significant pH change.

149 Typical band keratopathy in a 12-year-old girl with a long-standing history of juvenile rheumatoid arthritis and associated bilateral chronic uveitis. Note the classic distribution of the calcium deposits within the interpalpebral zone.

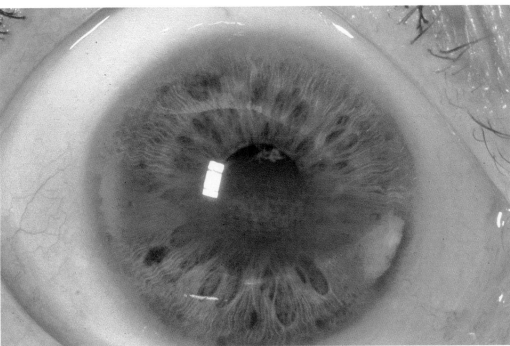

149

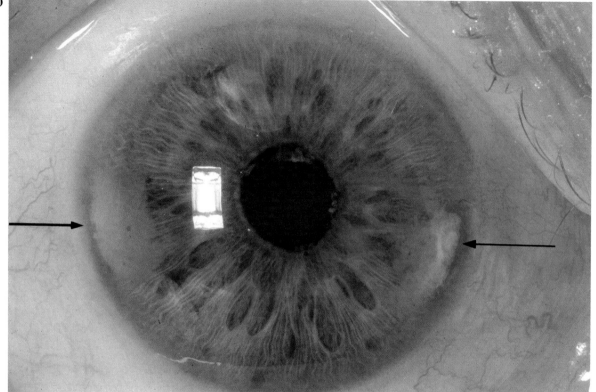

150 Early band keratopathy begins near the limbus, as seen here in the fellow eye of the patient in **149**. Note that calcium deposition has started within the interpalpebral fissure at 3 and 9 o'clock (arrows). Also visible is the sharp peripheral border, separated from the limbus by a clear interval. The central zone has not yet been involved.

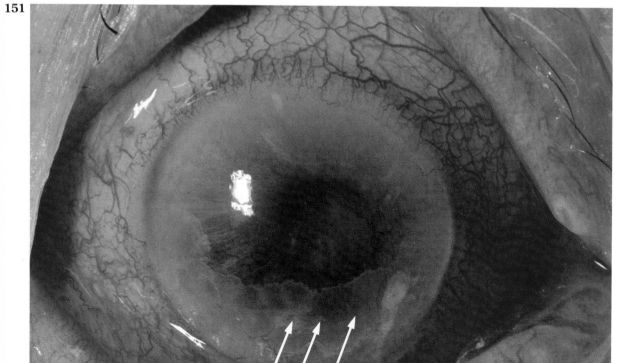

151 More advanced band keratopathy in a 65-year-old patient with neovascular glaucoma. Note the rubeosis iridis. There are clear, circular areas within the band (arrows), where corneal nerve endings penetrate Bowman's layer.

152 Prolonged use of pilocarpine drops, which contain the preservative phenylmercuric nitrate, was associated with the development of band keratopathy in this glaucoma patient.

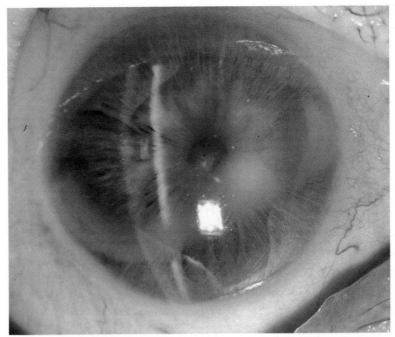

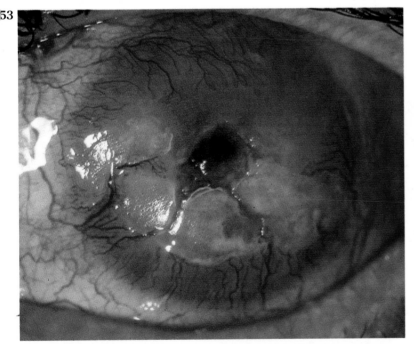

153 Alkali burns can lead to corneal vascularisation and severe calcific band degeneration, as seen in this 25-year-old patient who had suffered an alkali burn two years earlier. Note the large calcium plaques at the level of Bowman's layer.

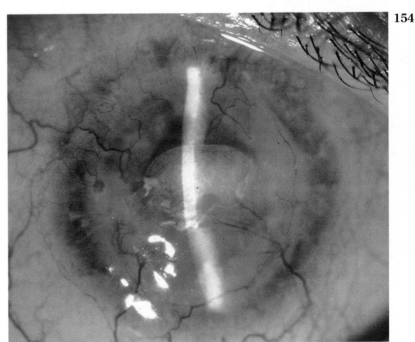

154 Band degeneration in a graft that failed after a rejection reaction. Note the central position of the deposits, and the clear periphery.

Calcareous degeneration

Unlike band keratopathy, calcareous degeneration involves the deeper corneal stroma as well as Bowman's layer. It is seen both in grossly distorted globes and in severe dry eyes with or without chronic ocular inflammation. Whereas most cases of calcareous degeneration have a gradual onset, the authors have recently reported cases (1991) in which calcium deposition developed rapidly over a period of a few days to a few weeks. Histopathological examination demonstrates that the most striking abnormality in these cases is the extensive, dense, granular calcification extending variably throughout the full thickness of the stroma, with secondary disturbance of the lamellar stromal architecture.

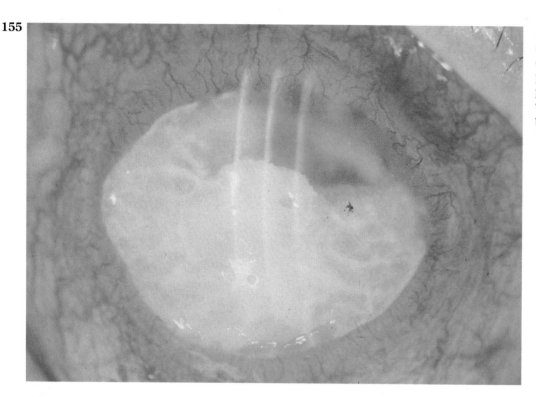

155 Triple slit-lamp beam examination of the right cornea of a 60-year-old patient with acute bilateral calcareous degeneration that had developed over a period of two weeks. The patient suffered from practolol-induced keratoconjunctivitis sicca. Full-thickness corneal calcification has involved 90% of the cornea, with a clear zone at the limbus.

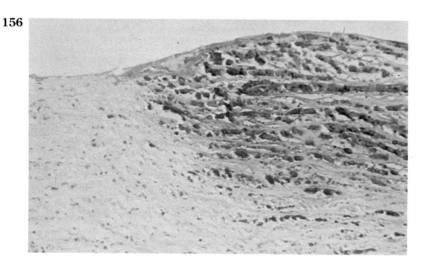

156 Light micrograph of the cornea shown in **155**, demonstrating extensive stromal calcification. This calcification was generally well circumscribed and confined to stroma-lacking epithelium. The lamellar architecture was mildly disturbed and a few keratocytes were seen to remain in the affected areas (Hematoxylin and eosin stain × 225). Transmission electron microscopy showed the granular calcification to consist of fine, needle-shaped crystals.

157 & 158 The fellow eye of the patient shown in **155**, demonstrating an acute progressive increase in the density of the calcific deposits. Note the corneal appearance at the time of presentation (**157**), and that two weeks later (**158**). This patient eventually underwent bilateral penetrating keratoplasty, with subsequent visual rehabilitation and no recurrence of the degenerative changes in the grafts.

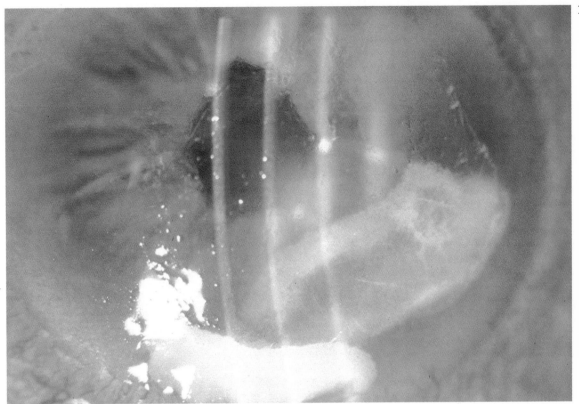

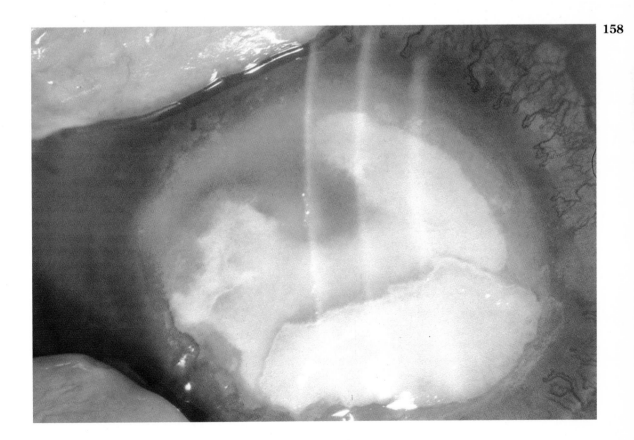

7 Pigmentary degeneration

Iron pigmentation

Iron deposition in the corneal epithelium can occur for a variety of reasons. It can be associated with conditions responsible for alteration of the shape of the cornea, which subsequently leads to disturbance of the pre-corneal tear film; pooling of the tears at certain areas results, followed by iron deposition. Iron pigment lines can occur in the form of Fleischer's ring at the base of the cone in keratoconus, the Stocker line at the head of a pterygium, the Ferry line around a filtering bleb, or in association with superficial scars (e.g. following radial keratotomy).

The most common iron pigment line, however, is the Hudson–Stähli line. Located at the junction of the middle and lower thirds of the cornea (at the line of lid closure), it extends horizontally, with a down arc in its centre. It may be single or double, or may split at the ends. This line is thought to be a degenerative age-related change, as its incidence increases with age.

Histological examination shows that the iron is deposited in the basal cells of the corneal epithelium. The source of the iron may be the perilimbal blood vessels; tear transferrin may help to carry it to its destination. Corneal iron lines cause no symptoms, and no therapy is required.

159 Iron pigment deposition in the corneal epithelium (arrows) developed in this 25-year-old patient nine months after radial keratotomy. Note the linear scars. The patient was asymptomatic and had an unaided visual acuity of 6/9.

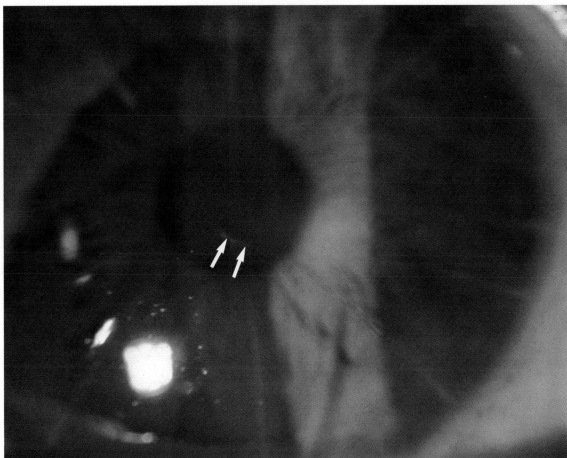

159

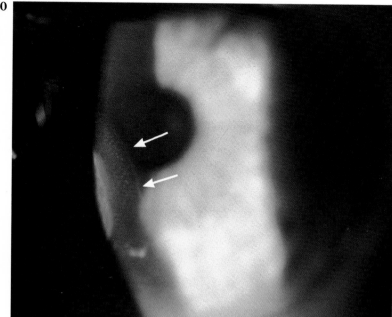

160 Stocker line: epithelial iron deposition in front of the advancing head of a pterygium (arrows).

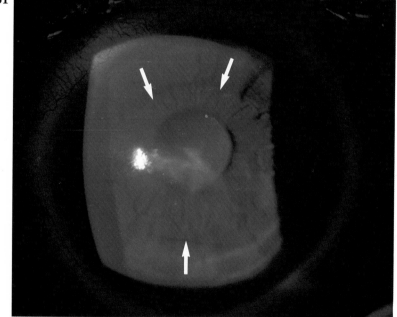

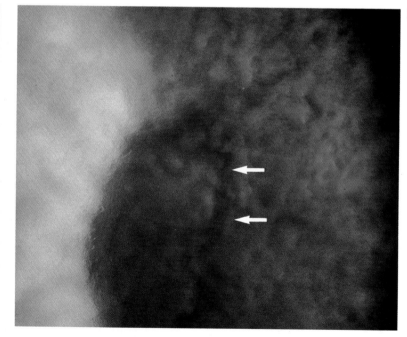

161 Fleischer's ring: iron has been deposited around the base of the cone in this 20-year-old keratoconus patient. The ring (arrows) is best seen by cobalt-blue illumination.

162 Hudson–Stähli line: most commonly occurring as an age-related degenerative change, it can also develop in young patients, in association with conditions that cause corneal surface irregularity. The pigment line (arrows) is here seen in a 29-year-old patient with Reis–Bücklers' dystrophy.

Blood staining of the cornea

Corneal blood staining is a serious degenerative change that occurs as a complication of traumatic hyphaema. It develops most commonly with secondary total haemorrhages in the anterior chamber with high or prolonged elevation of intraocular pressure. If the endothelial injury has been extensive, blood staining may occur with normal intraocular pressure. The blood staining may occupy the whole cornea or be localised to a small, central, disciform area. It appears as a rust-coloured opacity that changes with time through various shades of greenish black to grey. Clearing of the blood staining occurs from the periphery to the centre of the cornea, and in a posterior to anterior direction.

Histopathological examination reveals marked endothelial abnormali-ties, with a normal Descemet's membrane. Haemoglobin and erythrocyte breakdown products are found in extracellular and intracellular locations of the stroma, and there are degenerative changes in some keratocytes. The blood products are thought to penetrate through the discontinuous endothelium and the intact Descemet's membrane. The corneal opacity may take two to three years to clear, and results from the phagocytic action of the keratocytes and from the diffusion of haemoglobin breakdown products out of the cornea. However, in many cases, necrosis of the keratocytes occurs and the blood staining may be irreversible, indicating penetrating keratoplasty.

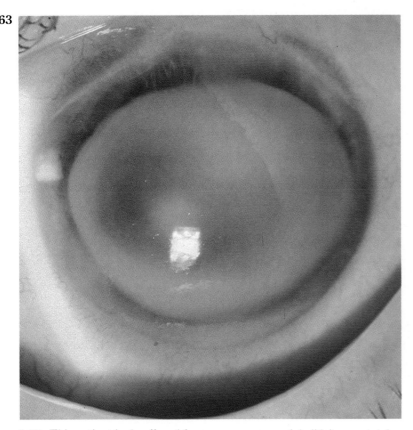

163 This patient had suffered from a severe squash ball injury; a total hyphaema resulted, with marked elevation of the intraocular pressure. Note that the hyphaema has resolved, leaving classic blood staining of the cornea. Note also the extent and the rusty red colour of the opacity.

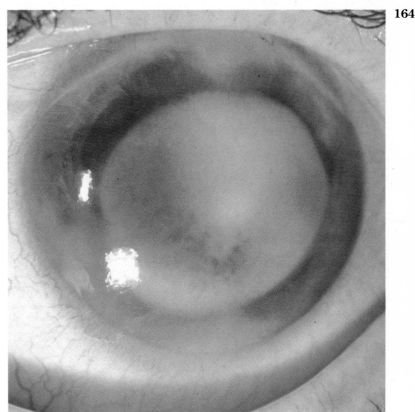

164 The same eye as shown in **163**, ten months later. Note the change in the colour, as well as the reduction in the size, of the opacity. Penetrating keratoplasty was eventually required for visual rehabilitation of the patient.

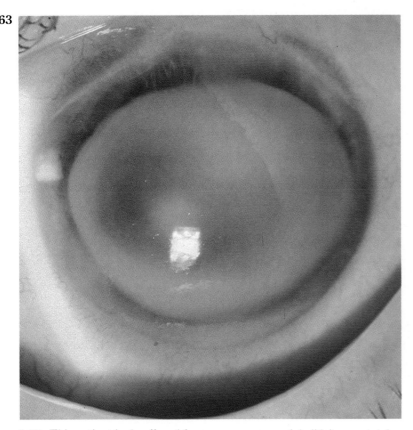

Vortex degeneration (corneal verticillata)

Vortex degeneration is a condition that used to be incorrectly described as 'vortex dystrophy'. In fact, it is a degenerative change caused by toxic keratopathy. It has been associated with amiodarone, choroquine, indomethacin, and chloropromozine therapy. A similar pattern is seen in Fabry's disease.

The corneal changes consist of whorl-like lines that appear to flow together in the infracentral corneal epithelium. These lines can be seen only on slit-lamp examination, and appear to consist of numerous, powdery, white or yellowish brown dots. It is believed that the vortex pattern is formed by the abnormal epithelial cells as they migrate towards the central cornea from the limbus.

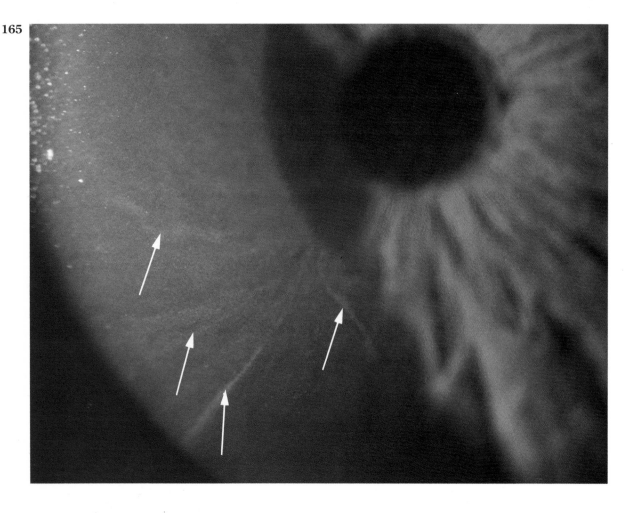

165 Corneal verticillata (arrows) developed in this 35-year-old woman after she had undergone chloroquine therapy for rheumatoid arthritis. Note the characteristic distribution of the typical whorl-like lines.

8 Lipid degeneration

Lipid degeneration is characterised clinically by the accumulation of a yellow or cream-coloured material in the corneal stroma. It can occur in two forms: primary or secondary. The latter is the most common form and is associated with a history of corneal inflammatory episodes with resultant stromal vascularisation. Certain diseases, such as herpes zoster keratitis, seem especially conducive to the development of lipid degeneration. The lipid infiltrates usually occur as an opacity in the corneal stroma, around an area of vascularisation. This dense, yellow-white opacity consists of discrete cholesterol crystals, together with neutral fats and phospholipids. The stromal lipid infiltrates may take the form of a circular disc or a fan-like arc around the ends of the vessels.

The primary form of lipid degeneration is usually bilateral. It occurs in the absence of any corneal neovascularisation or inflammation, and may be associated with a marked decrease in visual acuity.

166 Lipid degeneration developed in this patient with a history of recurrent herpes simplex keratitis and secondary corneal vascularisation. As the patient was asymptomatic and the stromal deposits did not progress to involve the visual axis, no treatment was required.

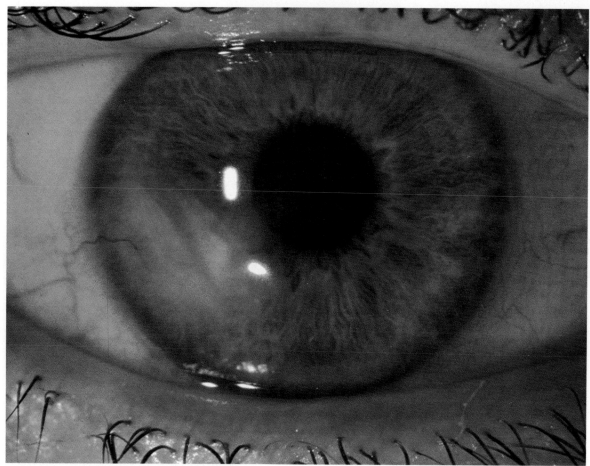

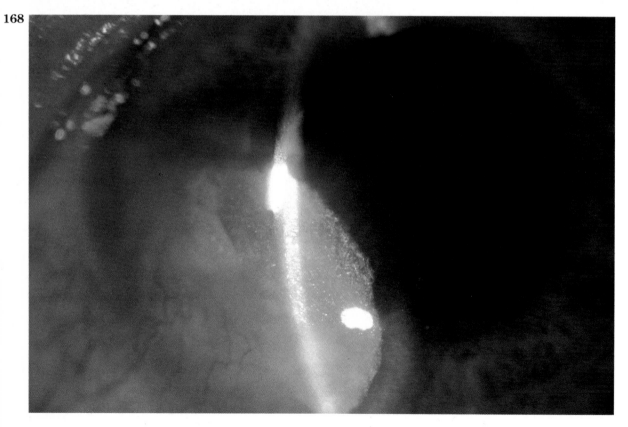

167 Herpes zoster keratitis is commonly followed by secondary lipid degeneration, as seen in this patient. The lipid deposits can be seen encroaching on the visual axis, with resultant impairment of vision.

168 Higher magnification of the lesion shown in **167** reveals the crystalline nature and midstromal location of the deposits.

169 Central lipid degeneration occurred in this 55-year-old woman after she had developed chronic exposure keratopathy related to an ipsilateral facial palsy. Note the associated corneal vascularisation and the circular shape of the opacity in the central stroma.

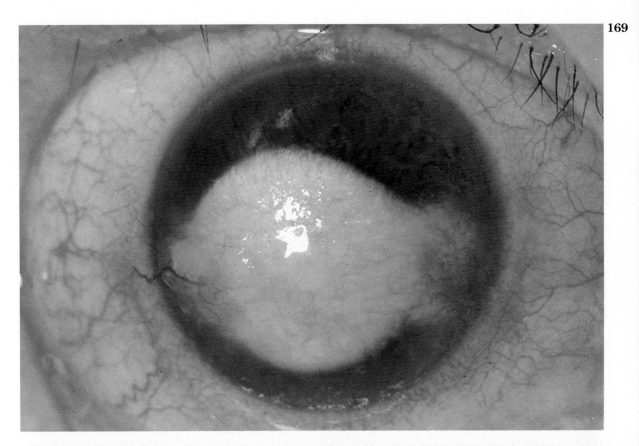

170 Localised, dense, peripheral lipid infiltrates occur if an arcus senilis is associated with pre-existing corneal or limbal vascularisation, as seen in this Asian woman. The patient had a history of trachoma with pannus formation.

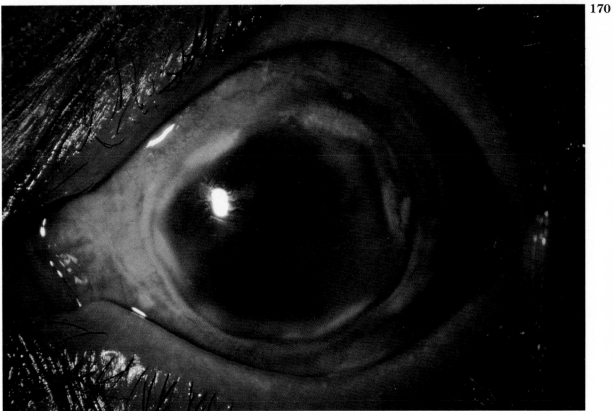

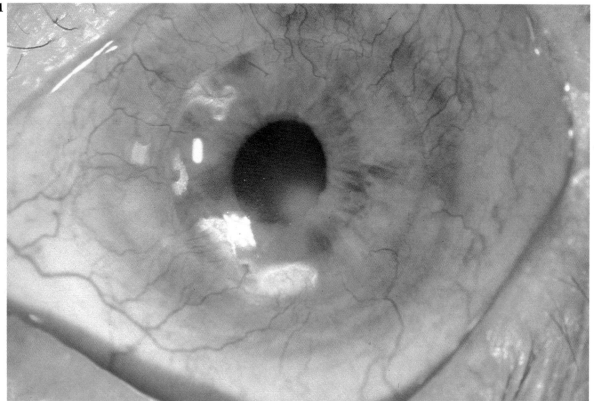

171 Lipid infiltrates may occasionally create a fan-like arc around the ends of abnormal vessels, as seen in this patient with a vascularised corneal transplant, performed following a chemical burn.

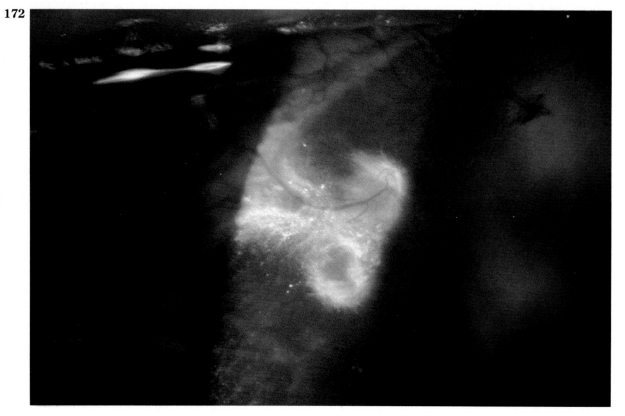

172 High magnification of the cornea shown in **171** clearly demonstrates the relation of the lipid infiltrates to the abnormal vessels crossing the graft–host junction.

9 Pterygium

Pterygium is a fibrovascular connective tissue overgrowth of the conjunctiva onto the cornea. It is usually triangular in shape, with a broad base on the nasal or temporal epibulbar surface and a blunted apex on the cornea. The pterygium has three components: the cap, which is the grey avascular zone that precedes the head of the lesion and surrounds it like a halo; the head, which is white and slightly elevated; and the body, which is a flat sheet of pink, highly vascularised connective tissue. When the pterygium is actively growing, the tissue is red and inflamed; as the lesion becomes inactive, vascularity diminishes and the redness disappears. Even in the fully developed form, a pterygium almost never involves more than one half of the cornea.

The pathogenesis of pterygia is unclear. The condition has been found to occur most frequently in populations living near the equator; the nearer to the equator, the greater the prevalence. The geographical distribution of pterygium and its anatomical location in the interpalpebral region both implicate the environment. The conjunctiva and the cornea absorb most of the infrared and ultraviolet radiation from sunlight, which can damage epibulbar tissue. The first sign of corneal invasion is a line of fibroblasts between the epithelial basement membrane and Bowman's layer. It seems that the fibroblasts follow this plane into the cornea, later guiding the bulky fibrovascular tissue along the same path. This invasion could be attracted by solar radiation-induced degenerative changes in the basal cell layer, or by an immunological response to altered basement membrane material.

Histologically, pterygia have changes consistent with solar elastotic degeneration of collagen. Bowman's layer eventually becomes fragmented, and the fibrovascular tissue of the pterygium head becomes firmly adherent to the superficial stroma over the sites of focal interruption in Bowman's layer.

Conjunctival malignancy, such as squamous cell carcinoma, and pseudopterygium must be included in the differential diagnosis of pterygium. A pseudopterygium can occur secondary to any peripheral corneal inflammation, such as marginal keratitis. It may also arise following chemical burns and cicatricial conjunctivitis. A pseudopterygium can be easily differentiated from a true pterygium by its lack of organisation into different components (i.e. cap, head, and body), by its atypical location, and by its lack of firm adhesion to the limbus.

The incidence of recurrence of pterygia following surgical excision is variable and depends upon the surgical technique, as well as upon the current environmental status of the patient. The authors' preferred approach to the management of a recurrent pterygium is superficial lamellar keratectomy followed by lamellar keratoplasty.

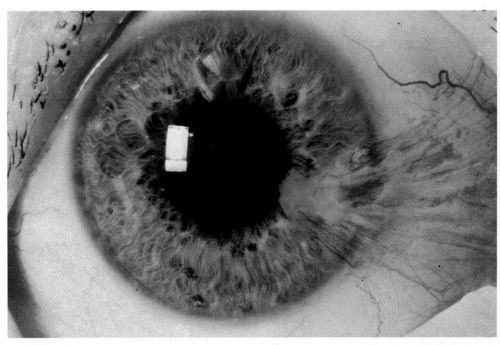

173 Actively growing pterygia develop more commonly in younger people, as seen in this 29-year-old man. This nasal pterygium has a typical triangular, fleshy appearance with a slightly elevated head. Examination of the degree of vascular dilatation in the bulk of the lesion and its leading edge reveals that the pterygium is active.

173

Components of the pterygium

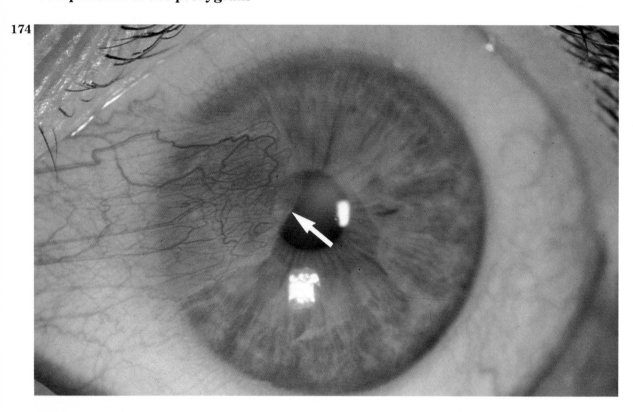

174 The head of the pterygium is firmly adherent to the cornea and is preceded by a grey zone, the cap, which is flat, avascular, and greyish white in colour.

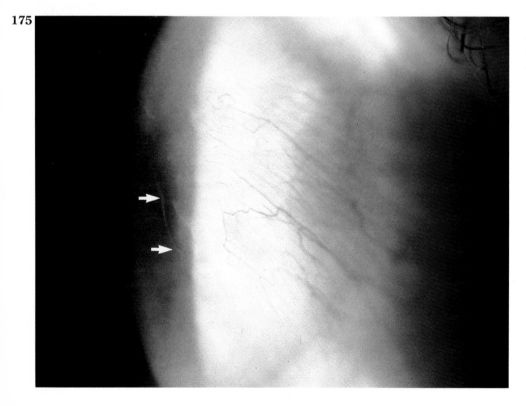

175 A Stocker line (arrows) is found in many cases of pterygium; it represents a line of iron pigment deposition in the epithelium bordering the corneal side of the head, i.e. preceding the grey zone.

176 The body of the pterygium is a fleshy sheet of pink, highly vascularised tissue. It is delineated from the normal conjunctiva superiorly and inferiorly by sharp folds. Unlike the firmly attached head, the body can be readily lifted from the underlying epibulbar surface. Note that the body is under horizontal tension, as evidenced by the vessels, which appear stretched and straight.

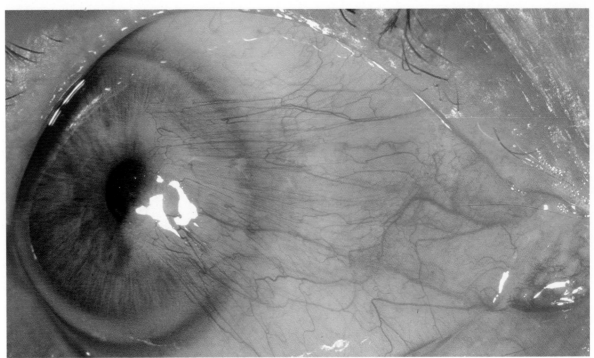

Recurrent pterygium

177 Pterygium recurred in this 35-year-old woman despite two previous excisions. Here the recurrence was associated with symblepharon formation between the body of the active lesion and the palpebral conjunctiva.

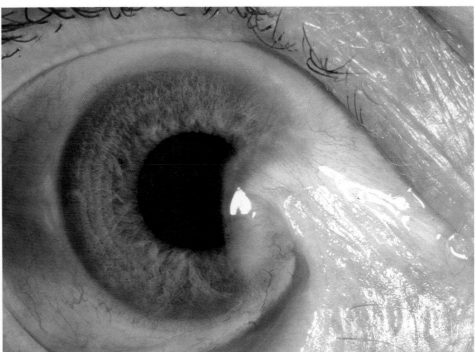

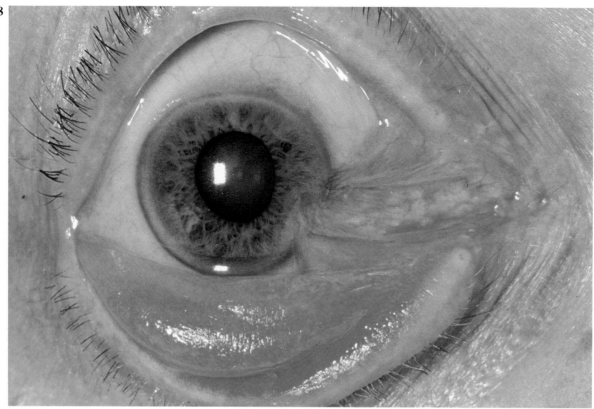

178 This patient was referred to the authors' unit, with history of recurrent pterygium despite five previous excisions. Note that the recurrent lesion has caused traction on the inner canthus structures, as well as secondary lower lid ectropion with conjunctival hyperaemia and keratinisation. The patient also suffered from diplopia on abduction, due to mechanical limitation of lateral gaze.

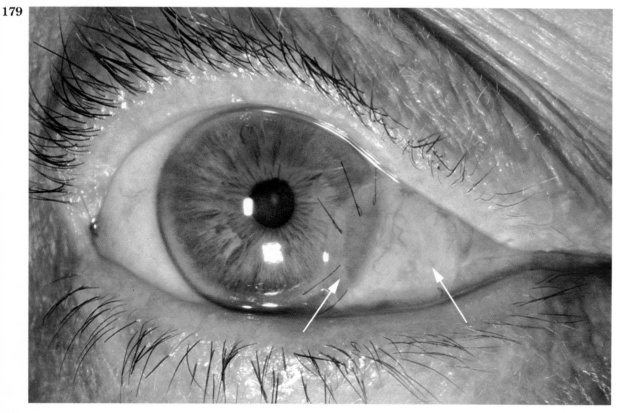

179 Postoperative appearance of the eye shown in **178** two months after a circular lamellar graft (arrows). Note the complete and spontaneous recovery of the lower lid to the normal position. The patient had no recurrence of the pterygium over a two-year follow-up period.

10 Salzmann's nodular degeneration

Salzmann's nodular degeneration is a gradually developing condition that appears in corneas with a previous history of chronic inflammation. The most common association is phlyctenular keratitis, followed by trachoma, vernal keratitis, keratoconjunctivitis sicca, and exposure keratopathy. However, a few cases may have lesions typical of Salzmann's nodular degeneration, but no history or clinical evidence of previous keratitis.

The disorder can occur at any age, but develops more frequently over the age of 50 years. The degeneration is bilateral in 80% of cases, and affects females more commonly than males.

The typical lesions present as bluish grey, elevated, fibrous nodular masses located in the superficial corneal stroma. The intervening cornea is clear, unless it has been involved through the pre-existing stromal scarring. The nodular lesions vary in number from one to nine, and are usually located in the midperiphery.

Light microscopy reveals evidence of pre-existing, old corneal inflammation, with scarring and vascularisation. The nodules, however, show no vessels or inflammatory cells. There is marked thinning of the epithelium overlying the nodules, and over these areas Bowman's layer is replaced by eosinophilic basement membrane-like material. The nodules show evidence of hyaline degeneration of collagen.

Although most cases are asymptomatic, some patients may complain of ocular irritation that is related to erosions of the epithelium overlying the nodules. Vision may also be impaired if the nodules are central. In such cases, lamellar or penetrating keratoplasty may be indicated.

180 In this 30-year-old woman, Salzmann's nodular degeneration developed in association with pre-existing corneal scarring caused by trachoma. The slit-lamp beam section (arrow) clearly demonstrates the surface irregularity caused by the nodule, and its anterior stromal location. Note that the nodule is situated at the junction of the scarred and the clear cornea.

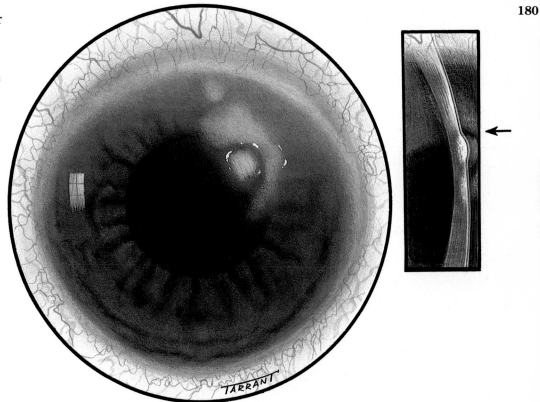

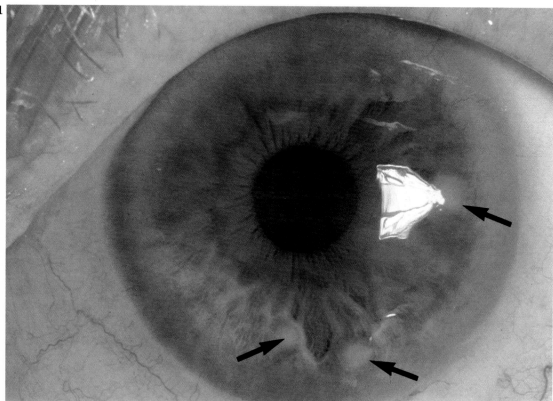

181 Between one and nine discrete lesions may arise in Salzmann's degeneration. This 45-year-old patient had three blue-grey nodules (arrows), with clear intervening stroma and no history of corneal inflammation. As the patient was asymptomatic, no treatment was required.

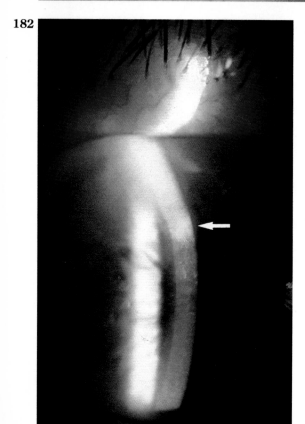

182

182 This patient developed Salzmann's degeneration following recurrent episodes of vernal keratitis. Note the anterior location of the nodule (arrow). His visual acuity worsened, and he complained of ocular irritation related to recurrent erosions of the epithelium overlying the nodule. Following lamellar keratoplasty, the patient became asymptomatic, with improvement of his visual acuity.

11 Spheroidal degeneration (climatic droplet keratopathy)

Spheroidal degeneration has been described with a variety of names including chronic actinic keratopathy, oil droplet degeneration, Labrador keratopathy, keratinoid corneal degeneration, elastoid degeneration, and Nama keratopathy. The incidence of the degeneration varies according to the geographical area, actinic exposure being the most likely basis for the differing geographical distribution. In addition to solar radiation, other factors related to the development of spheroidal degeneration include ageing, low humidity, corneal drying, and chronic exposure to wind, sand, or ice.

There are three types of spheroidal degeneration. Type I is the primary corneal form, which is bilateral, age-related, and not associated with other corneal diseases. Type II occurs secondary to climatic exposure and/or to pre-existing corneal disorders, such as traumatic corneal scarring, chronic corneal oedema, trachoma, and herpetic keratitis. Type III is the conjunctival spheroidal degeneration, which is associated with pinguecula in 86% of cases. In all three types, men are more frequently involved than women, in a ratio of 4:3, a fact that has been attributed to the greater outdoor exposure experienced by men.

The typical changes in climatic droplet keratopathy begin with the subepithelial accumulation of clusters of yellow or grey droplets that coalesce to form a band in the exposed area of the cornea. A clear zone may be identified between the deposits and the limbus in early cases, but this zone eventually becomes involved at a later stage. Three degrees of severity have been described: grade I, in which only the peripheral interpalpebral zone of the cornea is affected; grade II, in which the opacity spreads to the pupillary area, reducing vision to 6/36; and grade III, in which large, yellowish, opalescent nodules elevate the epithelium, reducing vision to less than 6/60.

Histologically, the corneal deposits are extracellular, and are composed of a proteinaceous material which appears as hyaline spheres in the anterior stroma and Bowman's layer.

Lamellar keratectomy or keratoplasty may be indicated in severe cases. The authors have also obtained good results with penetrating keratoplasty, with no clinical evidence of recurrence postoperatively. Excimer laser has recently proved to be very successful in the treatment of this condition, with no recurrence over a 12-month follow-up period.

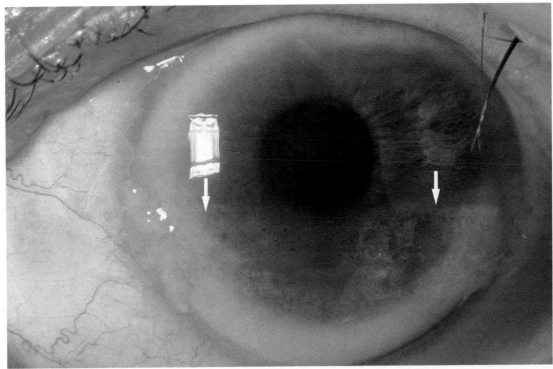

183 Bilateral climatic droplet keratopathy developed in this 55-year-old British woman who had been living in Africa for the previous 20 years. Note the typical band-shaped distribution of the yellowish droplets within the interpalpebral zone (arrows). The aggregates are larger and arranged in clusters at the nasal and temporal periphery.

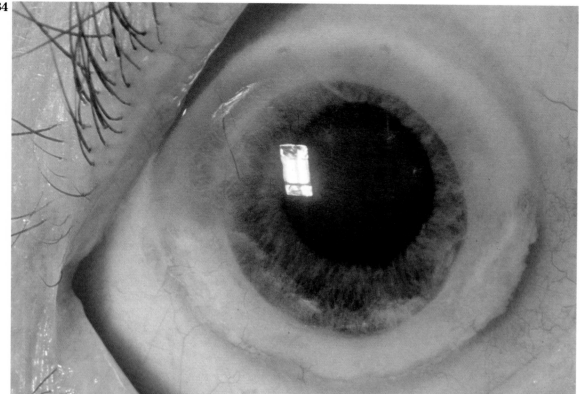

184 The fellow eye of the patient in **183**, five years after penetrating keratoplasty. Note the absence of any sign of recurrence in the donor cornea.

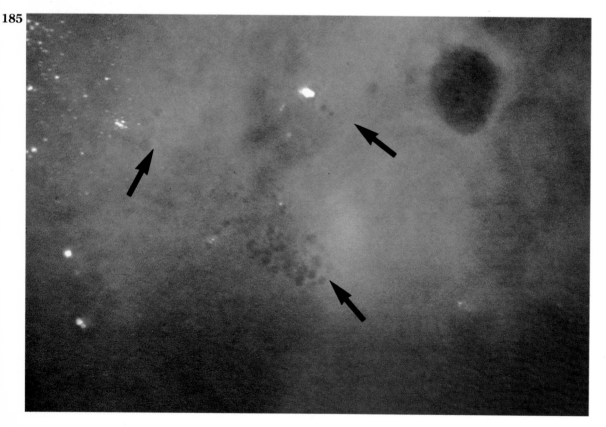

185 Secondary spheroidal degeneration (arrows) developed in the central cornea of this 45-year-old woman with a long-standing history of trachoma.

186 Spheroidal degeneration can occur on top of a pre-existing traumatic corneal scar, as seen in this patient (arrow). Note that, in contrast with the primary type, the degenerative changes in this case were localised to the area of corneal scarring; they did not assume a band-shaped configuration.

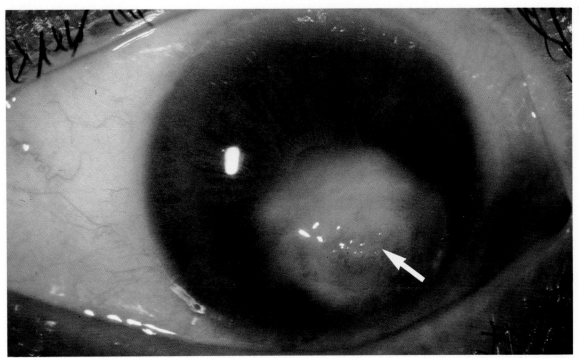

Histopathology of spheroidal degeneration

187 The corneal droplets appear as yellowish green, pleomorphic deposits that are located superficial and deep to Bowman's layer (arrow), and below in the anterior stroma (Van Gieson's stain × 40).

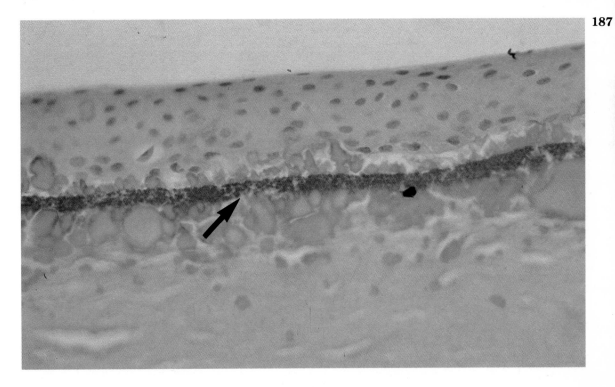

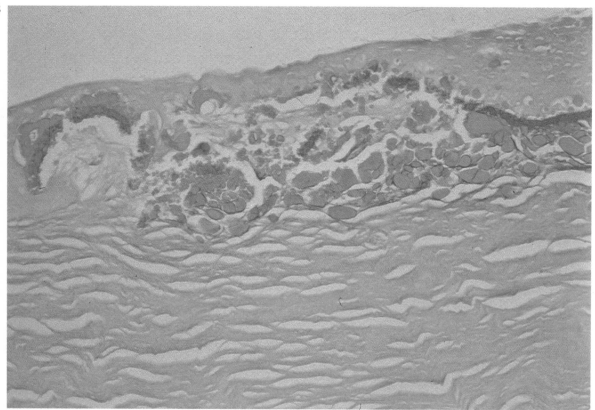

188 The large deposits visible in some areas have replaced a fragmented, degenerate Bowman's layer. Note the thinning of the epithelium overlying these areas. The deposits are extracellular and autofluorescent. The origin of the material forming these deposits may be proteins generated in the limbal conjunctiva, which diffuse into the corneal stroma and precipitate (Miller's elastic stain × 40).

12 Terrien's marginal degeneration

First described by Terrien in 1900, this marginal degeneration is bilateral in 86% of cases, and men are more frequently affected than women.

Terrien's marginal degeneration can occur at any age. It usually begins in the superior cornea, but may arise anywhere around the limbus. The earliest slit-lamp finding is a fine, punctate stromal opacity which is separated from the limbus by a clear zone. This is followed by superficial vascularisation of the involved area. As a result of the slowly progressive stromal thinning, a gutter develops parallel to the limbus. This gutter has a sloping peripheral edge and a sharp central edge. There is usually a characteristic line of lipid deposits at the central border of the lesion. The epithelium overlying the gutter is normal and does not stain with fluorescein. As the degeneration progresses, the thinned area may bulge ectatically. The gutter may spread circumferen-

tially in a direction parallel to the limbus, with the occasional development of pseudopterygium (20% of cases).

In most cases, the degeneration is a painless condition, the presenting symptom being progressive deterioration of visual acuity. This is related to corneal flattening in the involved area, which leads to high, often irregular, 'against the rule' astigmatism. However, in some young patients the condition may be associated with severe pain due to inflammation and necrosis of the peripheral cornea.

Light microscopy demonstrates subepithelial connective tissue and vessels with fibrillar degeneration of collagen.

No medical therapy has yet been effective in treating this condition. However, where there is impending or frank perforation, an annular lamellar or penetrating keratoplasty is indicated.

189 Terrien's marginal degeneration in a 35-year-old man with a history of painless, progressive deterioration of vision over a period of 15 months. The slit-lamp beam section clearly demonstrates the marked thinning of the superior cornea, with the associated secondary ectasia.

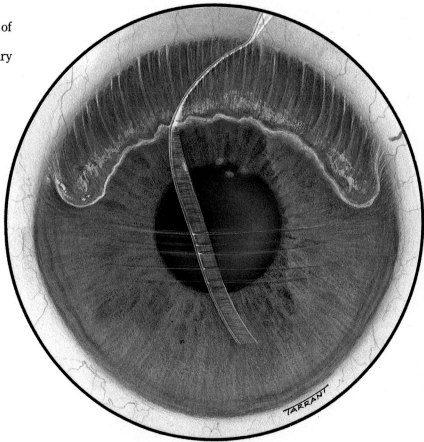

189

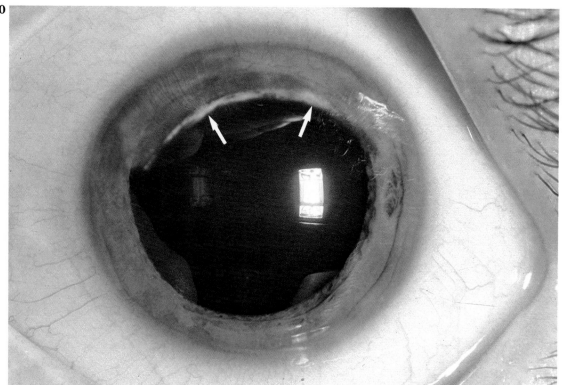

190 A typical superior gutter in a case of Terrien's marginal degeneration, demonstrating a sloping peripheral edge and a sharp central border which is highlighted by a white line of lipid deposits (arrows). These deposits come from the superficial vessels that invade the thin area from the limbus.

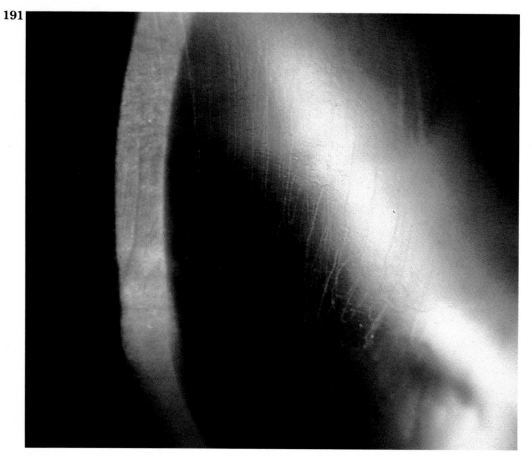

191 High-magnification slit-lamp photograph of the patient in **190**, showing the involved thin area of the cornea. Retroillumination clearly demonstrates the characteristic superficial vascularisation, which is formed by radial extension of vessels from the limbal arcades.

192 The fellow eye of the patient in **190**, showing a more advanced stage of Terrien's marginal degeneration. Note that the area of thinning has spread circumferentially, both laterally and medially, forming a gutter parallel to the limbus.

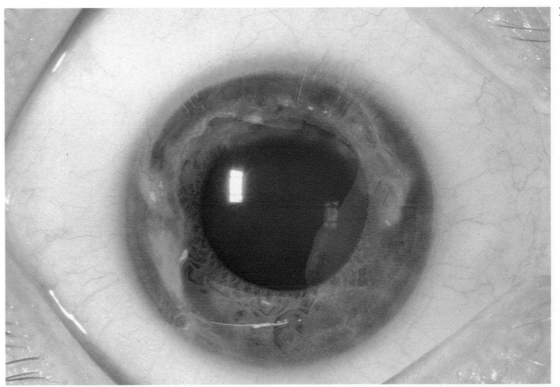

193 High-magnification triple slit-lamp beam in a 25-year-old patient with Terrien's marginal degeneration. Note the marked difference in corneal thickness between the involved superior thin area (long arrow) and the rest of the cornea (short arrow). The stretched superficial vessels in the thin area are clearly seen with retroillumination.

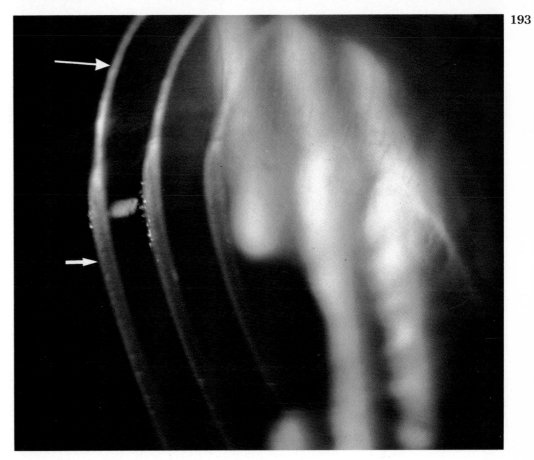

193

194 The same patient as in **193**. The authors have identified an interesting sign in patients who have advanced Terrien's marginal degeneration with secondary ectasia. In such cases, the involved cornea has a number of parallel, horizontal, subepithelial linear folds or striae, (arrows) which are located in the uninvolved part of the central cornea, below the ectatic area. It is believed that these lines are flexion folds caused by the marked flattening of the cornea in the vertical meridian, as they have been found to run parallel to the steep axis of the ectatic cornea.

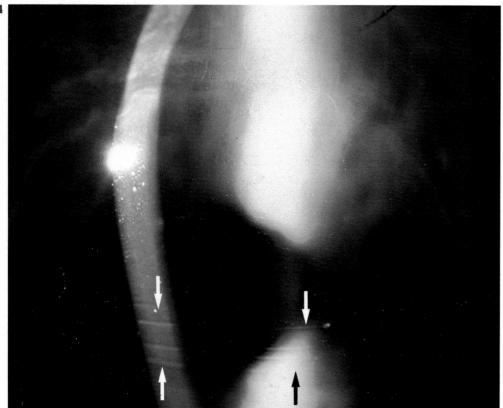

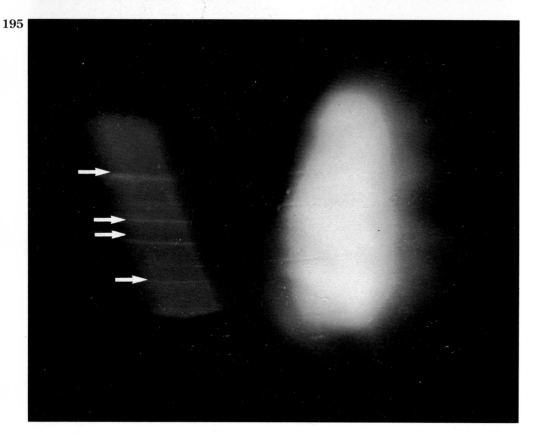

195 High-magnification slit-lamp photograph of the cornea shown in **194**, demonstrating the parallel, horizontal arrangement of the subepithelial folds. These folds and their anterior location are more clearly demonstrated in the illustration of this patient in **189**.

196 Keratoscope photograph of the case of advanced Terrien's marginal degeneration shown in **193 & 194**. Note the marked 'against the rule' astigmatism caused by flattening in the involved area. This patient had 10D of astigmatism, with the axis of the plus cylinder at 180°.

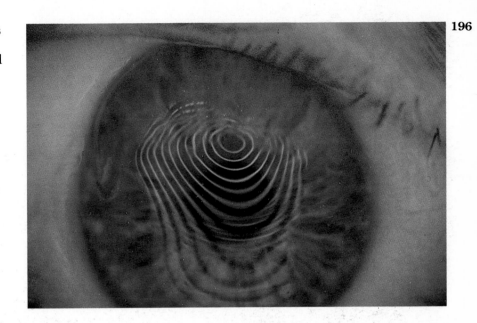

197 Perforation does not commonly occur in association with Terrien's marginal degeneration. However, in a few cases, perforation may either develop spontaneously in the area of thinning, or, as seen in this case, following minor blunt trauma. Note the iris prolapse at the site of perforation; an annular penetrating keratoplasty was performed to regain the structural integrity of the globe.

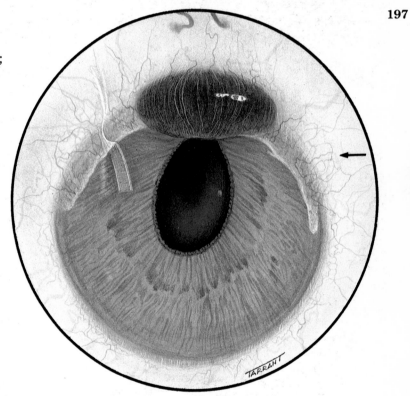

13 Pellucid marginal degeneration

Pellucid marginal degeneration is an uncommon ectatic corneal condition that usually presents between the second and fifth decades of life. It affects males and females equally, manifesting as an inferior corneal protrusion above a narrow band of clear, non-vascular, stromal thinning that is concentric to the inferior limbus. This band of thinning is between 1 and 2 mm in width, and there is usually an uninvolved area between it and the limbus. Acute hydrops may occur in the area of corneal thinning, secondary to breaks in Descemet's membrane. The corneal ectasia leads to flattening of the vertical meridian and 'against the rule' astigmatism that may be as high as 20 dioptres.

In contrast with Mooren's ulcer and Terrien's marginal degeneration, there is no lipid deposition or vascularisation. The condition can occur in conjunction with keratoconus in some patients, as described in several published reports. Histopathological examinations have been performed by four authors, and all agree that pellucid marginal degeneration may be a variant of keratoconus (Pouliquen, *et al.*, 1980; Rodrigues, *et al.*, 1981).

Hard contact lenses may be used when spectacle correction becomes ineffective, but in advanced cases, crescentic lamellar keratoplasty may be indicated.

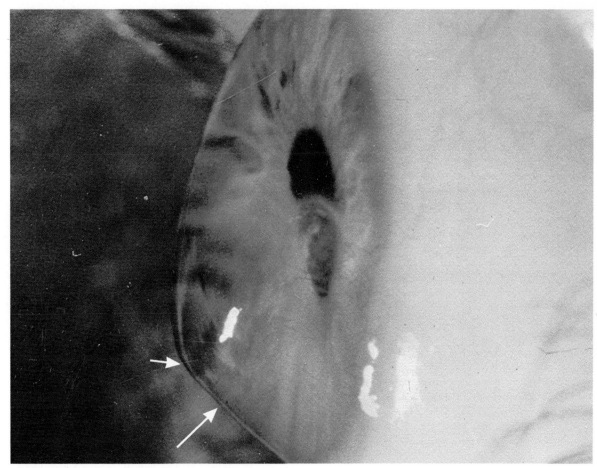

198 Pellucid marginal degeneration in a 40-year-old patient. Note the characteristic protrusion of the cornea (short arrow), which has developed above an inferior band of thinning situated 2 mm from the limbus (long arrow). This corneal change caused more than 15 D of central 'against the rule' astigmatism.

198

14 Corneal amyloidosis

Amyloidosis comprises a group of disorders characterised by the deposition of particular amorphous, eosinophilic, hyaline proteins in tissues. Amyloidosis can be primary or secondary, systemic or localised. Secondary systemic amyloidosis does not affect the cornea, and primary systemic amyloidosis does so only rarely.

Primary localised corneal amyloidosis is usually the result of direct extension from the conjunctiva, and can also involve the eyelids and the orbit. It presents as a soft, yellow, nodular thickening in the lids or conjunctiva. Treatment is by local excision. Lattice dystrophy may be considered as an autosomal dominant primary localised familial amyloidosis. A recessive form of corneal amyloidosis, which has been called 'gelatinous drop-like dystrophy', has been described in Japan.

Secondary localised amyloidosis of the cornea has been reported to occur following ocular trauma, trachoma, leprosy, chronic uveitis, keratoconus, and bullous keratopathy.

Depending on other associated factors, the cornea may be vascularised. The amyloid lesions appear as yellowish grey, fleshy, elevated, subepithelial masses. The clinical appearance of the lesions may be influenced by the primary disease.

The amyloid material in the cornea is identical to that present in other organs. It stains with Congo red, displaying birefringence and two-colour dichroism when viewed with a polarising microscope and green filter (*see* p. 27). Amyloid contains protein, carbohydrate, and polysaccharide components, as well as immunoglobulins.

Penetrating keratoplasty is indicated for secondary localised corneal amyloidosis only when vision is impaired. There is a high risk of rejection due to corneal vascularisation, and recurrences of amyloidosis in the graft are to be expected.

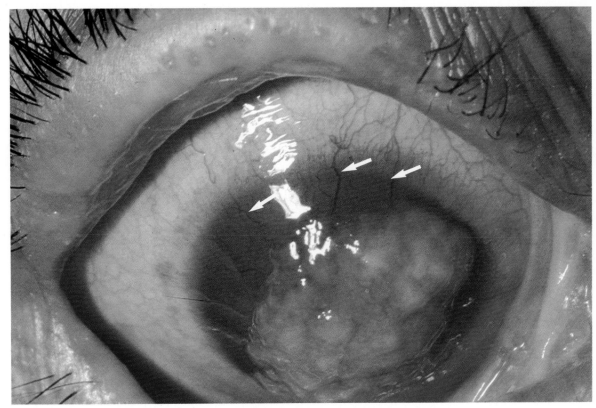

199 Secondary corneal amyloidosis in a patient with long-standing stromal and epithelial oedema due to Fuchs' dystrophy. Note the characteristic yellow-white, raised, fleshy masses, which create a nodular sur-face. Peripheral vascularisation (arrows) is commonly associated with secondary amyloidosis.

199

15 Superficial reticular degeneration of Koby

Koby described this rare, progressive, superficial corneal degeneration in 1927. The disorder is characterised by the appearance of a central white reticulum at the level of Bowman's layer. The epithelium, which becomes thickened, is speckled with a slightly brownish discoloration that provides a striking contrast to the white reticulum.

Following Koby's original case report, there was some doubt concerning the real existence of such a condition, as some authors suggested that Koby's case represented lattice dystrophy. However, further reports by Arguello, *et al.* (1950) and, more recently, by Perry and Scheie (1980), have confirmed that superficial reticular degeneration of Koby represents a distinct entity, which clinically resembles lattice dystrophy, but lacks a positive family history, severe visual loss, and the presence of recurrent epithelial erosions. Most patients repor-ted with this disorder are either middle-aged or have had long periods of chronic ocular inflammation.

Perry and Scheie suggested that this degeneration may represent an atypical form of band keratopathy. The white reticulum is formed by the atypical linear deposition of calcium salts at the level of Bowman's layer. The irregular, yellow-brown background tint is related to abnormal iron-pigment deposition in the basal epithelial layers, which probably occurs secondary to chronic disruption of the tear film. The brownish pigment extends just beyond the limits of the reticulum, and is unique to this corneal degeneration.

There may be progressive loss of vision in affected patients. However, visual acuity rarely deteriorates beyond 6/12.

200 Reticular degeneration of Koby in an eight-year-old boy with a history of bilateral chronic uveitis. Indirect illumination (scleral scatter) clearly demonstrates the fine, well-defined, reticular pattern involving the central cornea. The cornea of the fellow eye had an identical central reticular pattern (Courtesy of British Journal of Ophthalmology).

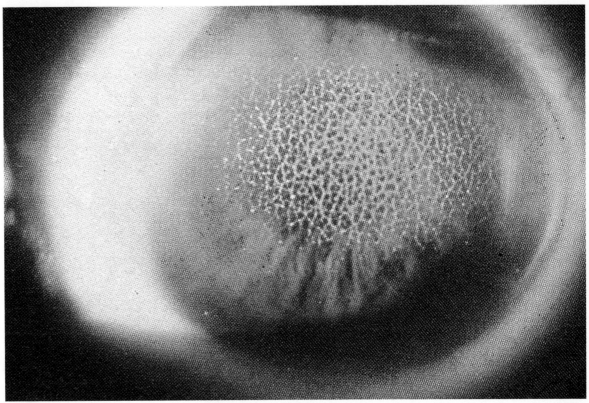

200

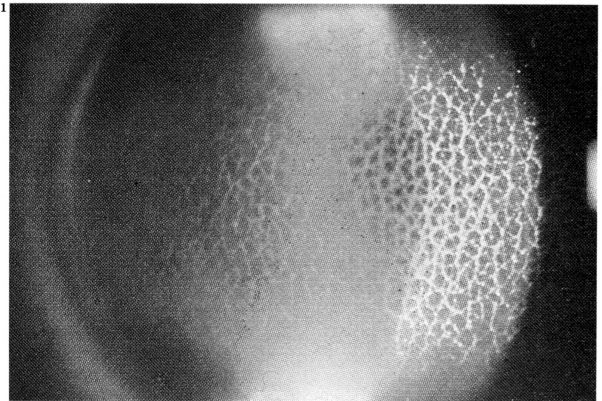

201 Broad oblique illumination demonstrates the superficial location of the reticulum at the level of Bowman's layer. Note that the opacities appear white with direct light, whereas with retroillumination, they appear light brown (Courtesy of British Journal of Ophthalmology).

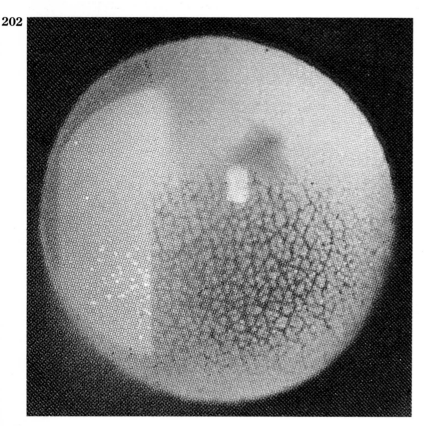

202 Retroillumination through a dilated pupil demonstrates the limits of corneal involvement. Visual acuity was 6/12 in both eyes.

Selected Reading

Abelson, M.B., *et al.* Recurrent keratoconus after keratoplasty. *Am. J. Ophthalmol.*, **90**: 672; 1980.

Akiya, S. and Brown, S. Granular dystrophy of the cornea. *Arch. Ophthalmol.*, **84**: 179; 1970.

Alexander, R.A., Grierson, I., and Garner, A. Oxytalan fibers in Fuchs' endothelial dystrophy. *Arch. Ophthalmol.*, **99**: 1622; 1981.

Aracena, T. Hereditary fleck dystrophy of the cornea. *J. Pediatr. Ophthalmol.*, **12**: 223; 1975.

Arentsen, J.J. and Laibson, P.R. Penetrating keratoplasty and cataract extraction. *Arch. Ophthalmol.*, **96**: 75; 1978.

Austin, P. and Brown, S.I. Inflammatory Terrien's marginal corneal disease. *Am. J. Ophthalmol.*, **98**: 189; 1981.

Bagolini, B. and Ioli-Spada, G. Bietti's tapetoretinal degeneration with marginal corneal dystrophy. *Am. J. Ophthalmol.*, **65**: 83; 1968.

Baum, J.L. Cholesterol keratopathy. *Am. J. Ophthalmol.*, **67**: 372; 1969.

Berkow, J.W., Fine, B.S., and Zimmerman, L.E. Unusual ocular calcifications in hyperparathyroidism. *Am. J. Ophthalmol.*, **66**: 812; 1969.

Berkowitz, P.J., *et al.* Presence of circulating immune complexes in patients with peripheral corneal disease. *Arch. Ophthalmol.*, **101**: 242; 1983.

Bourgeois, J., Shields, M.B., and Thresher, R. Open angle glaucoma associated with posterior polymorphous dystrophy. *Ophthalmology*, **91**: 420; 1984.

Bourne, W.M. Primary corneal endotheliopathy. *Am. J. Ophthalmol.*, **95**: 852; 1983.

Bourne, W.M., Johnson, H., and Campbell, J. The ultrastructure of Descemet's membrane. *Arch. Ophthalmol.*, **100**: 1952; 1982.

Boysen, G., *et al.* Familial amyloidosis with cranial neuropathy and corneal lattice dystrophy. *J. Neurol.*, **42**: 1020; 1979.

Bramsen, T., Ehlers, H., and Baggessen, L.H. Central cloudy corneal dystrophy of François. *Acta Ophthalmol.* (Copenh.) **54**: 221; 1976.

Broderick, J.D. Pigmentation of the cornea. *Ann. Ophthalmol.*, **11**: 855; 1979.

Broderick, J.D., Dark, A.J., and Peace, G.W. Fingerprint dystrophy of the cornea. *Arch. Ophthalmol.*, **92**: 483; 1974.

Bron, A. J. and Williams, H.P. Lipaemia of the limbal vessels. *Br. J. Ophthalmol.*, **56**: 343; 1972.

Bron, A.J., Williams, H.P., and Carruthers, M.E. Hereditary crystalline stromal dystrophy of Schnyder. *Br. J. Ophthalmol.*, **56**: 383; 1972.

Brown, A.C., Rao, G.N., and Aquavella, J.V. Peripheral corneal grafts in Terrien's marginal degeneration. *Ophthalmic Surg.*, **14**: 931; 1983.

Brownstein, S., *et al.* The elastotic nature of hyaline corneal deposits. *Am. J. Ophthalmol.*, **75**: 799; 1973.

Bücklers, M. Uber eine weitere familiare Hornhautdystrophie. *Klin. Monatsbl. Augenheikd.*, **114**: 386; 1949.

Burns, R.P. Meesmann's corneal dystrophy. *Trans. Am. Ophthalmol. Soc.*, **66**: 530; 1968.

Buxton, J.N. and Fox, M.L. Superficial epithelial keratectomy in the treatment of epithelial basement membrane dystrophy. *Arch. Ophthalmol.*, **101**: 392; 1983.

Buxton, J.N. and Lash, R.S. Results of penetrating keratoplasty in the iridocorneal endothelial dystrophy. *Am. J. Ophthalmol.*, **98**: 297; 1984.

Caldwell, D.R. Postoperative recurrence of Reis–Bücklers' corneal dystrophy. *Am. J. Ophthalmol.*, **85**: 577; 1978.

Caldwell, D.R., *et al.* Primary surgical repair of several peripheral marginal ectasias in Terrien's marginal degeneration. *Am. J. Ophthalmol.*, **97**: 332; 1984.

Curran, R.E., Kenyon, K.R., and Green W.R. Pre-Descemet's membrane corneal dystrophy. *Am. J. Ophthalmol.*, **77**: 711; 1974.

Fernandez–Sasso, D. and Acosta, J.E.P. Mulbran: Punctiform and polychromatic pre-Descemet's dominant corneal dystrophy. *Br. J. Ophthalmol.*, **63**: 336; 1979.

François, J. Heredo-Familial corneal dystrophies. *Trans. Ophthalmol. Soc. U.K.*, **86**: 367; 1966.

Maguire, L.J. and Meyer, R.F. Ectatic corneal degenerations. In: Kaufman, H., *et al. The Cornea*, pp. 485–510, Churchill Livingstone, New York, 1988.

Miller, A.C. and Krachmer, J.H. Epithelial and stromal dystrophies. In: Kaufman, H., *et al. The Cornea*, pp. 383–424, Churchill Livingstone, New York, 1988.

Moller, H.V. Interfamilial variability and interfamilial similarities of granular corneal dystrophy. *Acta Ophthalmol.* (Copenhagen), **67**: 667, 669; 1989.

Perry, H.D. and Scheie, H.G. Superficial reticular degeneration of Koby. *Br. J. Ophthalmol.*, **64**: 841–844; 1980.

Pouliquen, Y., Chauvand, E., Lacombe, E., *et al.* Degenerescence pellucid marginale de la cornée ou keratocone marginale. *J. Fr. Ophthalmol.*, **3**: 109; 1980.

Rodrigues, M.M., Newsome, D.A., Krachmer, J.H., *et al.* Pellucid marginal corneal degeneration: a clinico-pathological study of two cases. *Exp. Eye Res.*, **33**: 277; 1981.

Sharif, K.W. and Casey, T.A. Penetrating keratoplasty for keratoconus: complication and long-term success. *Br. J. Ophthalmol.*, **75**: 142–146; 1991.

Sharif, K.W., *et al.* Penetrating keratoplasty for bilateral acute corneal calcification. *Cornea*, **10** (6); 1991.

Smolin, G. Dystrophies and Degenerations. In: Smolin, G. and Thoft, R.A., *The Cornea*, pp. 427–455, Little, Brown and Company, Boston, 1987.

Sugar, A. Corneal and conjunctival degenerations. In: Kaufman, H., *et al. The Cornea*, pp. 441–459, Churchill Livingstone, New York, 1988.

Townsend, W.M. Pterygium. In: Kaufman, H., *et al.* The Cornea, pp. 461–483, Churchill Livingstone, New York, 1988.

Waring, G.O., Rodrigues, M.M., and Laibson, P.R. Corneal Dystrophies. I. Dystrophies of the epithelium, Bowman's layer and stroma. *Surv. Ophthalmol.*, **23**: 71; 1978.

Waring, G.O., Rodrigues, M.M. and Laibson, P.R., Corneal dystrophies. II. Endothelial dystrophies. *Surv. Ophthalmol.*, **23**: 147; 1978.

Index

Figures in italics refer to illustrations.